Ethical
Deliberation
in Multiprofessional
Health Care Teams

Ethical Deliberation
in Multiprofessional Health Care Teams

Edited by

Hubert Doucet
Jean-Marc Larouche
Kenneth R. Melchin

A project of the
Saint Paul University Centre
for Techno-Ethics

University of Ottawa Press

University of Ottawa Press gratefully acknowledges the support extended to its publishing programme by the Canada Council and the University of Ottawa.

We acknowledge the financial support of the Government of Canada through the Book Publishing Industry Development Program (BPIDP) for our publishing activities.

National Library of Canada Cataloguing in Publication Data

Main entry under title:

Ethical deliberation in multiprofessional health care teams

Includes bibliographical references.

ISBN 0-7766-0525-9

1. Medical ethics.   2. Chronically ill children—Care—Moral and ethical aspects.   I. Doucet, Hubert, 1938- II. Larouche, Jean-Marc, 1955-
III. Melchin, Kenneth R., 1949-

R729.5.H4E84 2001   174'2   C2001-901018-4

UNIVERSITÉ D'OTTAWA
UNIVERSITY OF OTTAWA

Cover illustration: *Entre deux solstices,* original drawing by Christiane Lemire. © 2000.

Typesetting: Christiane Lemire

ISBN 0-7766-0525-9

© University of Ottawa Press, 2001
  542 King Edward, Ottawa, Ont. Canada K1N 6N5
  press@uottawa.ca   http://www.uopress.uottawa.ca

Printed and bound in Canada

*To the memory of Edward Nolan,
friend and colleague at the Saint Paul University
Centre for Techno-Ethics*

Table of Contents

Introduction 9
    Hubert Doucet, Jean-Marc Larouche and Kenneth R. Melchin

Chapter 1   Historical Context: Deliberation and
    Methodology in Bioethics 13
    Hubert Doucet

Part 1 Implicit Ethics of Professionals in the Field of Pediatric Chronic Care

Introduction to Part 1 31
    Jean-Marc Larouche and Tim Flaherty

Chapter 2   The Nurse as Moral Agent 35
    Jean-Marc Larouche and Tim Flaherty

Chapter 3   The Physician as Moral Agent 57
    Jean-Marc Larouche and Tim Flaherty

Chapter 4   The Social Worker as Moral Agent 77
    Jean-Marc Larouche and Tim Flaherty

Chapter 5   Synthesis of Part 1 89
    Jean-Marc Larouche and Tim Flaherty

Part 2 Ethical Deliberation: Theoretical Perspectives from the Fields of Ethics and Conflict Studies

Introduction to Part 2 95
    Kenneth R. Melchin

Chapter 6   Theories of Discourse Ethics 97
    James Sauer

Chapter 7   The Cognitional Theory of Bernard Lonergan
and the Structure of Ethical Deliberation 113
Kenneth R. Melchin

Chapter 8   Value Conflicts in Health Care Teams 129
Peter Monette

Conclusion to Part 2 163
Kenneth R. Melchin

Part 3 Action Research: Ethical Deliberation in Multiprofessional Health Care Teams

Introduction to Part 3 169
Kenneth R. Melchin

Chapter 9   Action Research on Ethical Deliberation 171
Kenneth R. Melchin and Peter Monette

Chapter 10   Guide for Ethical Deliberation 187
*Peter Monette, Kenneth R. Melchin, Tim Flaherty,
Jean-Marc Larouche and Hubert Doucet*

Chapter 11   Thinking About Ethical Deliberation
in Multiprofessional Health Care Teams 199
Kenneth R. Melchin

Concluding Reflections 215
Kenneth R. Melchin

Appendix A Database for Documentary Analysis of Part 1 221

Appendix A Analytical Grid for the Action Research of Part 3 223

Appendix A Case Studies for the Action Research of Part 3 224

Bibliography 243

Introduction

Hubert Doucet,
Jean-Marc Larouche
and Kenneth R. Melchin

Technological changes have had a dramatic impact upon the financing, organization and delivery of health care services in Canada. Professionals and health care decision makers now wrestle with increasingly complex sets of challenges that must involve various types of professionals in programs of care. The result is that administrators, nurses, physicians, social workers and other professionals have had diverse roles to play in programs of care and, consequently, have insisted that their voices be heard in the decision-making process alongside the voices of patients and their families. Needless to say, the ensuing discussions have become difficult because the diverse professional perspectives have given rise to conflicts over the goals, strategies and institutional supports for patient care.

This study examines ethical deliberation in multiprofessional health care teams. While ethics typically focusses on the issues involved in patient care, we have placed the accent on the *dynamics of the deliberation process itself.* And while ethics frequently centres on issues explicitly identified as such, we have targeted values and aspects of professional ethos that *implicitly guide the deliberation process.*

To help understand ethical deliberation among diverse health care professionals, we have drawn upon resources from the analysis of health care professions, from ethical theory and from the field of conflict resolution. These resources have been synthesized into a set of tools for understanding and guiding ethical deliberation in health care teams. To illustrate the relevance of these tools for health care teams, we have carried out a case-study observation of two teams of professionals working in the field of pediatric chronic illness.

Two sets of hypotheses inform this work. First, despite the work of hospital ethics committees, most ethical decisions on patient care are made outside of this structure, often in the health care units themselves. Furthermore, when professionals in these units gather to make decisions involving ethical issues, discourse and decision making are often influenced by the hierarchical or institutionalized relationships among the various professions. Finally, the self-understanding of each professional often carries a set of implicit values that shapes the deliberation process without being articulated openly and evaluated critically in the discussions of the team.

Second, when conflicts arise among professionals in health care teams, team members often turn to ethicists for their expertise in resolving issues. To offer such expertise, ethicists need tools for analyzing the dynamics of the deliberation process as well as tools for analyzing the issues. Furthermore, the ethical issues are often so closely bound up with the professional and technical aspects of the case that ethicists make their best contribution by developing tools for use by the professionals themselves.

Guided by these hypotheses, this study examines the ethical deliberation process and proposes tools to help teams of professionals in their own effort to wrestle with the issues. The overall goals are: (1) to investigate how professionals experience value conflicts and make decisions on ethical issues in cases where their diverse forms of involvement bring diverse ethical perspectives into the team discussions; and (2) to develop tools for ethical deliberation that could help professionals in the team discussion and decision making.

To meet these goals, the study is divided into three parts. Part 1 is a documentary analysis of literature related to professionals involved in health care teams. We have focussed, in particular, on professionals typically involved in pediatric chronic care. However, the issues arising in the analyses are sufficiently general that the insights developed here are relevant to a variety of health care contexts. The goal in this part is to establish a typology of the implicit ethics of the principal professions involved in the team deliberations: nurses, physicians and social workers.[1] A study of each profession reveals a number of diverse professional types, each with its own cluster of implicit values. Insights into these implicit values allow researchers and practitioners to anticipate forms of ethical conflicts that can arise from the interaction among diverse types.

Part 2 deals with the process of ethical deliberation, and here we review published literature from the fields of conflict studies and ethical theory. The goal throughout this section is to draw on resources from conflict studies and theoretical ethics to develop analytic tools for studying

---

1.   The choice of these professions is explained in the Introduction to Part 1.

ethical deliberation in health care teams. The overall theoretical framework for the analysis comes from the philosophy of Bernard Lonergan.

Part 3 takes the results of parts 1 and 2 into an action-research case-study analysis of ethical deliberation in multiprofessional health care teams. The researchers observed two teams of health care professionals involved in the field of pediatric chronic care working through a series of prepared case studies. Their deliberations are analyzed using analytical tools developed from parts 1 and 2. On the basis of the observations drawn from these analyses, a *Guide for Ethical Deliberation* is presented to help practitioners deal with the ethical aspects of cases encountered in the deliberation among professionals in health care teams. The guide is presented in chapter 10 of this study. Part 3 concludes with an extended reflection on how the diverse parts of the project fit together within the overall framework provided by the cognitional theory of Bernard Lonergan. And we suggest lines for further research that could build upon this work and test the empirical validity of its findings.

To set the background for the study and to situate it within the context of alternative approaches in bioethics, an essay on "Deliberation and Methodology in Bioethics" has been included, in chapter 1. And the study concludes with a brief résumé of the findings.

This volume has been a collaborative effort. The editors of the volume and directors of the project are Hubert Doucet,[2] Jean-Marc Larouche[3] and Kenneth R. Melchin of the Centre for Techno-Ethics at Saint Paul University, Ottawa, Canada. However, the success of the project is due, in no small measure, to the two research assistants responsible for overseeing the work of the project, Peter Monette and Tim Flaherty. Two members of the research team, James Sauer and Kevin Murphy, contributed to sections in this volume. Finally, we must recognize the excellent contributions of the members of the research team: Jean-Eudes Charbonneau, Kathryn Howe, Nancy Lepage, Jean-Louis Munn and Melissa Trono of the Centre for Techno-Ethics.

We greatly appreciate the gracious support and cooperation of Vicki Bennett of the University of Ottawa Press. She was most helpful in guiding us through the review and publication process and has been a constant source of encouragement.

Strategic subsidies in applied ethics received from the Social Sciences and Humanities Research Council of Canada (SSHRC) made it possible for researchers at the Centre for Techno-Ethics to undertake and

---

2. Hubert Doucet is currently director of the Bioethics Program at the Université de Montréal.

3. Jean-Marc Larouche is currently professor in the Département des sciences religieuses at the Université du Québec à Montréal.

bring to completion two research projects in the field of health care ethics for the chronically ill.[4] This volume presents the results of the work of the second of these projects, "Ethical Deliberation in the Field of Pediatric Chronic Illness." We are grateful for the work of the Council in supporting innovative lines of research in ethics.

Finally, we are indebted to Saint Paul University for providing financial assistance at a number of points along the way of this project. The university provides ongoing financial support for the Centre for Techno-Ethics and has provided special financial assistance for the editing and publication of this volume. In particular, our thanks go out to Michel Bergeron, Director of Research Services, who has done everything possible to ensure the publication of this volume.

---

4.   The first project is "Technology and Chronic Illness: An Ethical Challenge" (SSHRC no. 806-91-0014). The report of this project is entitled "Parameters for Ethical Reflection and Responsible Action in the Field of Chronic Illness." This first report introduces the problem of ethical deliberation in discourse among diverse professionals and it sets the stage for the development of the goals and the structure of the second project, "Ethical Deliberation in the Field of Pediatric Chronic Illness" (SSHRC no. 806-92-0027).

Chapter 1

Historical Context: Deliberation and Methodology in Bioethics

Hubert Doucet

The revival of interest in ethical issues concerning biomedicine and health care in the mid-sixties was undoubtedly a search for meaning. Not only was it a protest against certain types of experimentation on human subjects, it also represented a desire to make medicine a more humane enterprise. Whatever interpretation the ethical project of the time took—for example, Van Potter and André Hellegers developed different approaches to bioethics—the revival was oriented toward a promotion of the kind of medicine that is moral.

In this search for meaning, methodological issues could not be avoided. On the contrary, they were an essential facet of the ideal envisaged by the initial players in this revival. In 1970, the field was dubbed "bioethics," a name that represents one of its essential features, interdisciplinarity. The method was seen as an essential part of the nature of the enterprise. The Social Sciences and Humanities Research Council of Canada, in its 1989 report *Towards a Canadian Research Strategy for Applied Ethics*, confirms this interpretation. One of the main goals of the revival was to bring together people of different intellectual horizons to discuss major issues related to the development of biomedicine.

In the first part of this paper, I will highlight some facets of the interest in methodological issues raised at the origin of the bioethical movement. In the second part, I will focus on methodologies of the decision-making process that have been developed in order to help individuals or groups make a decision when faced with difficult problems. In the third part, I will explain the reasons behind our group working toward new or different avenues in the area of moral decision making.

METHODOLOGICAL ISSUES AT THE ORIGIN OF BIOETHICS

Bioethics, by definition and understood in a broad sense, is inter-disciplinary. It is clear when looking at the origin of the term that it was coined with a view to bringing two worlds that normally ignore one another into dialogue. As early as 1971, Van Potter, from the Wisconsin Medical School at Madison, Wisconsin, claimed that he had "invented a new word and a new scholastic enterprise called *Bioethics*" defined as "the combination of 'biological knowledge and human values.'"[1] *Bio* represented the science of living systems and *ethics* the knowledge of human value systems. His goal was to "build a bridge between the two cultures of science and the humanities."[2] In the same year, André Hellegers established and directed, at Georgetown University in Washington, the Kennedy Institute of Ethics, which included a Center for Bioethics. He "believed that bioethics would be a unique discipline combining science and ethics."[3] As early as 1968, he had invited the Protestant moral theologian Paul Ramsey to spend the first of two semesters at the Georgetown University Faculty of Medicine in order to generate dialogue with physicians concerned with ethical dimensions of their work.[4] According to Warren Reich, Hellegers could also be considered the father of the expression "bioethics."

Hellegers and Potter challenged the classical tradition of grounding ethics in the disciplines of philosophy and theology. Inspired by the work of Aldo Leopold, Potter developed a more comprehensive vision for bioethics that would draw upon the disciplines of evolutionary biology, ecology and cybernetics. His goal was to merge science and philosophy into a new discipline, "bioethics." Hellegers' vision would be to put the accent on a dialogue among diverse fields of research and scholarship as well as different life experiences. As he indicated in an interview in 1979, his was a truly ecumenical approach.

In 1973, Daniel Callahan, the founder of the Hastings Center, wrote an article entitled "Bioethics as a Discipline." The article "authenticated and registered in the appropriate academic chronicles the birth of the word 'bioethics' and the discipline that bore the name."[5] In his text, Callahan

---

1.   Van R. Potter, "Bioethics for Whom?" *Annals of the New York Academy of Sciences* 196 (1972): 201.

2.   Warren T. Reich, "The Word 'Bioethics': Its Birth and the Legacies of Those Who Shaped Its Meaning," *Kennedy Institute of Ethics Journal* 4 (1994): 321.

3.   Reich, "The Word 'Bioethics,'" 323.

4.   Paul Ramsey, *The Patient as Person* (New Haven, Conn.: Yale University Press, 1970), xix-xx.

5.   Reich, "The Word 'Bioethics,'" 331.

stated that a good methodology needs to "display the fact that bioethics is an interdisciplinary field in which the purely 'ethical' dimensions neither can nor should be factored out without remainder from the legal, political, psychological and social dimensions."[6]

If there was agreement that interdisciplinarity was the most appropriate methodological approach, the structure and the requirement of the method were never totally elucidated. For example, Callahan, on the one hand, entitled his 1973 article "Bioethics as a Discipline," and throughout the text refers to "a discipline to be shaped," a discipline that "is not yet burdened by encrusted traditions and domineering figures."[7] On the other hand, the discipline is described as interdisciplinary. He mentions "the interdisciplinary work of bioethics," "frustrating interdisciplinary session"[8] and "the fact that bioethics is an interdisciplinary field."[9] The conclusion of the article has the same ambiguity that is highlighted above. Indeed, one wonders what exactly "interdisciplinary" means here. Does it refer to a field of knowledge in which various individuals, coming from different horizons, participate? Or does it represent an individual, a bioethicist, who is required to possess all the qualities of the specialists in the various disciplines making up bioethics? A good training in bioethics

> requires, ideally, a number of ingredients as part of the training—which can only be life-long—of the bioethicist: sociological understanding of the medical and biological communities; psychological understanding of the kind of needs felt by researchers and clinicians, patients and physicians, and the varieties of pressures to which they are subject; historical understanding of the sources of regnant value theories and common practices; requisite scientific training; awareness of and facility with the usual methods of ethical analysis as understood in the philosophical and theological communities—and no less a full awareness of the limitations of those methods when applied to actual cases; and, finally, personal exposure to the kinds of ethical problems which arise in medicine and biology.[10]

---

6. Daniel Callahan, "Bioethics as a Discipline," in *Biomedical Ethics and the Law*, ed. J. M. Humber and R. F. Almeder (New York: Plenum Press, 1976), 9.

7. Callahan, "Bioethics as a Discipline," 4.

8. Ibid., 7.

9. Ibid., 9.

10. Ibid., 10.

These remarks could be interpreted to mean a bioethicist alone would bear the responsibility of interdisciplinarity. Other texts indicate a different position. They recognize that "interest in bioethics has involved a broad coalition of specialists from the sciences, the humanities, and the social sciences."[11] In a 1988 interview, Daniel Callahan remembers his own evolution: "As I discovered the broader domain of medical ethics, I realized the need for a new interdisciplinary field: no existing field had a monopoly on this area."[12] In the mid-seventies, with the development of the field and its professionalization, Callahan came to fear that interdisciplinarity itself could be jeopardized.[13] However, if the author authenticated the term "bioethics," his 1973 methodology did not clearly promote dialogue among the individuals involved in the various disciplines at play when decisions needed to be made.

Two explanations can help us understand why his position was ambiguous. They also underline the challenge of interdisciplinary work in bioethics. With a background in philosophy, Callahan may have assumed that bioethics is subsumed under one of the already participating disciplines.[14] This parallels the position of leading scholars of that period who would concur with a statement Danner Clouser made in 1978: "Bioethics is not a new set of principles or maneuvers, but the same old ethics being applied to a particular realm of concerns."[15] In a study made on the methods employed by some leading writers in the field of bioethics, Ronald Green found that where methodology is concerned, "both medical ethics and the somewhat broader field of bioethics ... are not usually distinguished."[16] In that sense, bioethics remains a discipline, as the title of Callahan's 1973 article indicates. How could the field be termed "interdisciplinary" if the central and unique method of bioethics is philosophy?

The second way Callahan's position is ambiguous is that his analysis does not take into account the peculiar combination of disciplines involved.

---

11. Daniel Callahan, "The Emergence of Bioethics," in *Science, Ethics and Medicine: The Foundations of Ethics and Its Relationship to Science*, vol. 1, ed. H. T. Engelhardt and D. Callahan (New York: The Hastings Center, 1976), xvii.

12. Daniel Callahan, "An Interview with Daniel Callahan," *Second Opinion* 9 (1988): 55.

13. Callahan, "The Emergence of Bioethics," xviii.

14. Corinna Delkeskamp, "Interdisciplinarity: A Critical Appraisal," in *Knowledge, Value and Belief*, ed. H. T. Engelhardt and D. Callahan (New York: The Hastings Center, 1977), 330.

15. K. Danner Clouser, "Bioethics," in *Encyclopedia of Bioethics*, vol. 1 (New York: The Free Press, 1978), 116.

16. Ronald M. Green, "Method in Bioethics: A Troubled Assessment," *The Journal of Medicine and Philosophy* 15 (1990): 180.

Usually, the practice of interdisciplinarity is a dialogue among sciences, and not sciences with philosophy. As mentioned by Corinna Delkeskamp:

> While philosophy allows one to address explicitly the ethical implications of scientific knowledge as applied to society, the participation of philosophy as a discipline different in kind seems to suggest an inequality in the interdisciplinary cooperation.[17]

One of the most interesting attempts to define the method of interdisciplinarity was made by Maurice de Wachter in 1979 in an article published first in French and rewritten in 1982 under the title "Interdisciplinary Bioethics: But Where Do We Start?"[18] For the author, interdisciplinary bioethics is a dialogue between researchers of different disciplines, not a substitute for the competencies and responsibilities of traditional disciplines. Indeed, "interdisciplinarity puts all disciplines in a wider perspective, and new tasks and responsibilities are added to previous ones." This is achieved through different phases *each of which mark specific efforts and contributions by participants of various disciplines.*"[19] This approach is what makes bioethics different from traditional medical ethics, in that the former is born from the need "to manage a hold of what is now escaping the grasp of many disciplines working separately."[20] De Wachter puts the emphasis especially on the first step, which he calls "methodical epochè": "from experience, we know that omitting such original epochè bars the road of interdisciplinarity."[21] The author borrows the term "methodical epochè" from the language of philosophy. It is a matter of suspending, as with Descartes, the methodical doubt. For de Wachter, it means that the participants of the interdisciplinary work will, as a first step, suspend their disciplinary reading of the situation. Its role is to set "a stage within which the total issue becomes visible to all participants."[22]

At its outset, bioethics is clearly defined as interdisciplinary. Robert Morison claimed that its greatest achievement is "to have shown the academy that interdisciplinary scholarship really is possible."[23] Originally,

---

17. Delkeskamp, "Interdisciplinarity," 331.

18. Maurice de Wachter, "Le point de départ d'une bioéthique interdisciplinaire," in *La bioéthique, Cahiers de bioéthique*, no. 1 (Quebec: Les Presses de l'Université Laval, 1979), 103-116; reprinted in Maurice de Wachter, "Interdisciplinary Bioethics: But Where Do We Start?" *The Journal of Medicine and Philosophy* 7 (1982): 275-287.

19. de Wachter, "Interdisciplinary Bioethics," 279.

20. Ibid., 283.

21. Ibid., 284.

22. Ibid., 286.

23. Robert S. Morison, "Bioethics After Two Decades," *Hastings Center Report* 11 (April 1981): 9.

bioethics was mostly seen as a dialogue between biological sciences, social sciences and humanities. But the field was soon transformed. There has been a "very rapid movement of these issues from the realm of theory and speculation into the real world, particularly into the world of courtrooms and legislatures."[24] The changes transformed the methodological approach, so that the developments of the field were to work against the interdisciplinary strategy.[25]

FROM FOUNDATIONAL CONCERNS TO APPLIED ETHICS

From foundational issues, the bioethical discussion moved to practical decision making. There were, as just mentioned, decisions made in courtrooms and legislatures. But also new participants began to be involved in the process: they were health care professionals, such as physicians, nurses and social workers; chaplains working at the bedside; and outsiders, such as ethicists, lawyers and administrators. They met in research ethics committees, known in Canada as research ethics boards (REBs) and in the United States as institutional review boards (IRBs), and in hospital ethics committees. The new context "tended to overpower some of the earliest interest in the deeper speculative and foundational side of the questions."[26] Emphasis put on practical decision making highlighted new methodological concerns.

Due to the new context, bioethics soon became similar to biomedical ethics and medical ethics, and thus was interpreted as a form of applied ethics.[27] The latter will have to face three major methodological issues. A first issue is related to the fact that biomedicine challenges the "naturally given." Dilemmas arise as a result of our increased control over the process of reproduction and dying. The decisions become more and more complex. A second issue is related to the fact that decisions have to be made in a context that has become pluralistic. The pluralism is ideological not only in the sense that there is no consensual philosophy or common religion,

---

24. Callahan, "An Interview," 56.

25. Morison, "Bioethics After Two Decades," 9.

26. Callahan, "An Interview," 56.

27. There are numerous debates over the meaning of the term "applied ethics." In relation to bioethics, see Barry Hoffmaster, "The Theory and Practice of Applied Ethics," *Dialogue* 30 (1991): 213-234; Edmund Pellegrino, "Bioethics as an Interdisciplinary Discipline: Where Does Ethics Fit in the Mosaic of Disciplines?" in *Philosophy of Medicine and Bioethics*, ed. R. A. Carson and C. R. Burns (Dordrecht: Kluwer Academic Publishers, 1997), 1-23; Hubert Doucet, "La bioéthique, des fondements philosophiques cachés," in *Les Annales du vivant* (Paris: Presses Universitaires de France, 1999), 914-915.

but also in the sense that various actors in the health care field now claim that they must have a voice in the decision-making process. Finally, ethics is seen as a practical enterprise. Decisions have to be made and efficient processes have to be sketched in order to come to decisions that will be applicable. Practically speaking, applied ethics is a tension between two forces, the principles to be applied and the case to be solved.

The Role of Principles

In 1973, the American government established the National Commission for the Protection of Human Subjects of Biomedical and Behavioral Research. Its mandate, based on its inauguration, was to set policies that would "emanate not just from the medical profession, but from ethicists, theologians, philosophers and many other disciplines."[28] Among the important reports published by the Commission was *The Belmont Report*, which had a major influence in determining the method to be used in biomedical applied ethics. The method was based on principles. Three were proposed. The first, which is respect for persons, incorporates at least two fundamental ethical considerations: respect for autonomy and protection of persons of impaired or diminished autonomy. Second is the ethical principle of beneficence, which refers to the ethical obligation to maximize benefits and minimize harms. This latter aspect of beneficence has come to be known as non-maleficence. The third is that of justice, which obligates one to treat each person in accordance with what is morally right and to give each individual his or her due.[29]

Since 1979, these principles have been largely adopted in the United States, Canada and elsewhere in Western countries and international organizations. Tom Beauchamp and James Childress, in their very influential work *Principles of Biomedical Ethics*, published the same year, added a fourth principle: non-maleficence.[30] These four were by then known as "the principles of bioethics." That the *International Ethical Guidelines for Biomedical Research Involving Human Subjects* from the Council for International Organizations of Medical Sciences (CIOMS) borrowed the formulation of their principles almost textually from *The Belmont Report* without mentioning the fact demonstrates that these principles have become

28. Edward Kennedy, quoted by David J. Rothman, *Strangers at the Bedside* (New York: Basic Books, 1991), 188.

29. National Commission for the Protection of Human Subjects of Biomedical and Behavioral Research, *The Belmont Report: Ethical Principles and Guidelines for the Protection of Human Subjects of Research* (Bethesda, Md.: The Commission, 1979), 4-10.

30. Tom L. Beauchamp and James F. Childress, *Principles of Biomedical Ethics* (New York: Oxford University Press, 1979).

commonly accepted. These *Guidelines* state that "all research involving human subjects should be conducted in accordance with three basic principles, namely respect for persons, beneficence and justice."[31] The "principlism" has been so well accepted that Danner Clouser and Bernard Gert have compared the role played by the "principles of biomedical ethics" approach to a kind of ritual:

> Throughout the land, arising from the throngs of converts to bioethics awareness, there can be heard a mantra "beneficence ... autonomy ... justice..."[32]

Why have Beauchamp and Childress built bioethics on these four principles? In the foreword of the first edition of *Principles of Biomedical Ethics*, the authors explain their perspective. The four moral principles they present should apply to a wide range of biomedical problems such as abortion, euthanasia, behaviour control, research involving human subjects and the distribution of health care. These principles connect the various dilemmas that biomedicine faces. The objective is to overcome a lack of methodology in biomedical ethics: "such a disjointed approach often relies on the discussion of cases, with little attention to the principles that both create and illuminate the dilemmas."[33]

On the other hand, in pluralist societies, it is recognized that individuals and groups do not share the same philosophical system or ethical theory. If in a moral philosophy principles are justified, according to these authors, by ethical theories, what is the theory that justifies the four principles of bioethics? In fact, the proponents of these principles "claim to derive principles from several different theories, none of them they judge to be adequate" and "there is no attempt to show that the different theories from which the principles are presumably derived can be reconciled."[34] A theory of bioethics could not even have been envisaged in a political society committed to pluralism. It could be said that, due to the various moral systems, the strategy has consisted in avoiding discussion of a possible theory to call for second-level principles that could achieve more consensus. It would be the only approach that would make difficult case solving possible. If there is no theory of bioethics, there is a practice that appeals to principles.

---

31. Council for International Organizations of Medical Sciences (CIOMS), *International Ethical Guidelines for Biomedical Research Involving Human Subjects* (Geneva: CIOMS, 1993), 10.

32. K. Danner Clouser and Bernard Gert, "A Critique of Principlism," *The Journal of Medicine and Philosophy* 15 (1990): 219.

33. Beauchamp and Childress, *Principles of Biomedical Ethics*, vii.

34. Clouser and Gert, "A Critique of Principlism," 232.

An Implicit Methodology

How do these principles work? Based on my own experience with different hospital ethics committees, I would like to describe the "methodology" used by these committees in making case consultations; it is a four-step method. It is not a formal methodology but rather an implicit one. In this, I want to highlight how members of ethics committees aspire to objectivity and strive for consistency in their procedures. My experience agrees with the description we find in the literature.

The first step could be described as fact finding. It consists in gathering relevant information. After a presentation of the situation, which is usually made by a physician and completed by other members of the health care team, members of the ethics committee ask for more information. Establishing the medical facts and then the psychosocial facts helps them understand the issues at stake in the situation. In this investigative phase, I have noticed different attitudes in members of hospital ethics committees. Some members remain unsatisfied with the information received. They ask for more and more medical information as if the addition of knowledge would make the appropriate answers appear. Others take another approach. For them, the medical factors tend to silence the psychosocial factors; they make us lose sight of the patient. The questions of this second group attempt to address the lack of real situational information about the context of the patient. A third group looks for a better global understanding of the medical and psychosocial elements in order to build an overall balanced picture.

A second step consists in identifying the moral or ethical issues at stake. What exactly is the problem under consideration? Is it a dilemma created by the development of modern medicine? A clash of values between a patient and health care professionals? A conflict between different groups of professionals? A disagreement between a patient and his or her family? Is it a request from a patient or his or her family that the team has to face for the first time and that creates a certain uneasiness and uncertainty? Two elements need to be highlighted. The problem raised has a name in terms of medical ethics. Categories such as informed consent, truth telling, euthanasia, futility of treatment and so on help members of ethics committees structure their thinking amid the multiplicity of information. The second element is related to the various readings made by the different individuals involved in the case; ethics committees are faced with conflicts of interpretation. It is in this context that the principles enter the conversation.

In the third step, the principles will be applied to the bioethical problems. They will be used as guides for thinking through the dilemmas. The case will show, for example, that some members focus more on the principle of beneficence; they want the good of the patient, as medicine defines it. Other participants in the team put the emphasis on the patient's autonomy: a competent patient's wishes should have priority over a physician's opinion. But what should happen if a competent patient requests a futile treatment that will deprive another patient of useful treatments? In this case, should justice prevail over autonomy? What if a patient requests euthanasia? In such a situation, does respect for a physician's values not override a patient's autonomy? Most of the time, the discussions reveal sharp conflicts between these principles.

"What to do?" involves a fourth step. At times, the ordering of principles will lead to negotiations and compromise. At other times, the choice of one principle over another will be seen as the most appropriate foundation for the recommendation. In the North American context, the principle that will most often be privileged is autonomy, with informed consent as its corollary. Whatever the final recommendation (which depends on the singularity of the case), the principles serve as a reference to show that the advice is objectively based.

In numerous sessions or courses on health care ethics and decision making that I have given to physicians, health care administrators and civil servants in public health, I have seen the same model develop. When principles of bioethics have been commonly accepted, they normally give rise to similar patterns of thinking about moral issues in the field of health care. Moreover, such an ethical workup is "analogous to the clinical makeup of a diagnostic or therapeutic problem."[35] However, this method is not without major limitations.

The first critique to be addressed to the method I have presented is that there is no place for the members of the health care team or the patient and his or her family to make sense of their situation. The actors have been eliminated.[36] The different steps lead to interpreting cases through the spyglass of conflicts of values, so that the facts are subsumed under the principles that will determine the decision. The situations are usually far more complex. When patients, families or health care team members come to an ethics committee, it does not take long to discover that their case is, in fact, a story in which certain moral feelings of an individual, some professional sensitivity of another individual or an important ethical value of a third is profoundly challenged by others. It is not only an intellectual conflict about interpretation of values or principles. The meaning and the orientation of a person's life or commitment are at stake. Principlism ends up being a reductionist approach.

---

35. Edmund D. Pellegrino, "The Metamorphosis of Medical Ethics: A 30-Year Retrospective," *JAMA* 269 (1993): 1160.

36. Barry Hoffmaster, "The Theory and Practice of Applied Ethics," *Dialogue* 30 (1991): 218.

The objectivity of the approach tends to obscure the complexity, the richness and the contradictions of the case. This is the second critique. The history of the patient, the experience of his or her illness, and his or her relationship with family members or significant others are not the focus of attention. There are, on the one hand, the medical facts and, on the other hand, the psychosocial facts. Often, both factors are interpreted as opposing one another: what the patient requests goes against the ability of medicine or what nurses are asking of physicians sounds irrational to the latter. The method promotes a dualistic approach. This is why it is often said that the clash of values is rather a conflict between reason or objectivity, on the one side, and emotion or subjectivity, on the other. A further analysis would show that the clash is between two interpretations of reason, one which could be called rational and the other contextual. Principlism does not allow for a reflection that could integrate all the dimensions of the situation.

A third critique could be addressed to the method. It is assumed that the different participants in the discussion interpret the four principles in the same manner. Are they not objective principles? It is presupposed that the dilemmas that have been identified are identically understood by the various participants since the principles are the same. But, in fact, participants do not interpret these principles in the same way. Beneficence as understood by physicians is often quite different for a nurse or a patient. To prolong a life could be seen as the beneficent obligation of a physician while a nurse would consider it her duty to stop treatment in the name of the same principle. This could explain why nurses who are so vocal in claiming that there are major ethical issues in their different units are silent in case consultations at an ethics committee. The concepts that are used do not correspond to their interpretation. The clash would also be a clash of language among the participants.

These different critiques correspond to the critique that is presently addressed to principlism. We have seen new directions in bioethics emerge that counteract the trend of the principle approach. Some could be considered reinterpretation, radical or not, of these principles,[37] while others

---

37. Among authors who could be mentioned here are Edmund D. Pellegrino and David C. Thomasma, *A Philosophical Basis of Medical Practice: Toward a Philosophy and Ethic of the Healing Professions* (New York: Oxford University Press, 1981); William F. May, *The Physician's Covenant: Images of the Healer in Medical Ethics* (Philadelphia: Westminster, 1983); Mark Siegler, "Clinical Ethics and Clinical Medicine," *Archives of Internal Medicine* 139 (1979): 914-915; Norman Daniels, *Am I My Parents' Keeper? An Essay on Justice Among the Young and the Old* (New York: Oxford University Press, 1988); Daniel Callahan, *What Kind of Life: The Limits of Medical Progress* (New York: Simon and Schuster, 1990).

really are new directions.[38] The debates around the foundations of bioethics are also debates about methods.

TOWARD NEW AVENUES IN ETHICAL DELIBERATION

It is in this context that our project has been elaborated. Having been involved for years in long-term health care institutions, with ethics committees and also with health care teams, I had come to the conclusion that the methodology used within the context of applied ethics had major shortcomings. First, it did not correspond to real-life situations in the sense that it turned away from the story of the patient. Second, it did not meet the needs of the various participants in the deliberations. Following a previous research project we had undertaken, we decided to focus the present one on the second aspect of the shortcomings, knowing very well that we could be criticized for not being patient-centred. We decided to look more carefully at *ethical deliberation in multiprofessional health care teams*. In this way, we wanted to look more precisely at the way professionals proceed in their decision making and to propose methodological tools that would help them integrate a patient's narrative in their deliberation.

A first objective of the new research project was to examine how conflicts of an ethical nature are lived and how decisions are made in long-term care units. For practical purposes, we chose pediatric units. The particular situation of children who are hospitalized in these units causes conflicts among the different professionals involved in the care of these patients. Moreover, the relations between these professionals and the parents are often tense. Each professional has his or her personal values and, at the same time, develops a sense of responsibility in accordance with the culture and the ethics of his or her own professional group. The hierarchical organization and the division of labour are added factors that determine the decision-making process. This explains why the discussion among members of a health care team may be heated; ethics opens a door

---

38. Among authors who could be mentioned here are those who reintroduce virtue ethics or casuistry and those who propose a feminist ethics, an ethics of care or narrative ethics. James F. Drane, *Becoming a Good Doctor: The Place of Virtue and Character in Medical Ethics* (Kansas City, Mo.: Sheed and Ward, 1988); Albert R. Jonsen and Stephen S. Toulmin, *The Abuse of Casuistry* (Berkeley: University of California Press, 1988); Susan Sherwin, *No Longer Patient: Feminist Ethics and Health Care* (Philadelphia: Temple University Press, 1992); M. Leininger, "Caring: A Central Focus of Nursing and Health Care Services," *Nursing and Health Care* 1 (1980): 135-143; Rita Charon, "Narrative Contributions to Medical Ethics," in *A Matter of Principles? Ferment in U.S. Bioethics*, ed. E. R. Dubose, R. P. Hamel and L. J. O'Connel (Valley Forge, Pa.: Trinity Press International, 1994).

leading to discussion of other issues. At times, an ethicist is called into the consultation to help solve the dispute. The different levels of complexity in the case and the various levels of tension among the members of the health care team are such that the ethicist is often required to play the role of mediator. In this context, our team wanted to examine more closely the way in which decisions of an ethical nature are made in pediatric long-term care units.

Our second objective was to elaborate, propose and evaluate a guide of deliberation in view of helping health care teams in their decision making. To regularly call on ethics committees to solve difficult issues faced by health care teams runs the risk of making ethics a technocratic tool. We believe that health care teams should be qualified to integrate the ethical component into their clinical decisions, even in the most difficult cases. However, teams need methodological support in order to achieve this goal. In the field of health care ethics, consensus has become a central area of concern. Dialogue and conflict management are seen more and more as a key element of the ethical process[39] but they only begin to be critically examined in order to highlight its implications, strengths and limits.[40] The development of methods of discussions has not been a real concern in the field of health care ethics. However, such methods are needed in order to allow health care teams to make decisions that would take into account the various facets to be considered in complex and difficult cases. They are especially needed in the domain of pediatric chronic illness. Indeed, long-term care in pediatrics is paradigmatic of the difficulties with which technological developments confront modern medicine.

In order to achieve these objectives, our conceptual approach had to be different than the principled approach I have described. A proposal

---

39. Joseph L. Allen, *Love and Conflict* (Nashville: Abington, 1984); Jürgen Habermas, *Communication and the Evolution of Society* (Boston: Beacon Press, 1979); Paul Ladrière, "De l'expérience éthique à une éthique de la discussion," *Cahiers internationaux de sociologie* 88 (1990): 43-68; Thomas Ogletree, *Hospitality to the Stranger* (Philadelphia: Fortress, 1985); Mary Beth West and Joan McIver Gibson, "Facilitating Medical Ethics Case Review: What Ethics Committees Can Learn from Mediation and Facilitation Techniques," *Cambridge Quarterly of Healthcare Ethics* 1 (1992): 63-74.

40. Anne Fagot-Largeault, "La réflexion philosophique en bioéthique," in *Bioéthique: Méthodes et Fondements*, ed. Marie-Hélène Parizeau (Montreal: ACFAS, 1988), 3-16; Mildred Z. Salomon et al., "Toward an Expanded Vision of Clinical Ethics Education: From the Individual to the Institution," *The Kennedy Institute of Ethics Journal* 1 (September 1991): 225-245; Robert M. Veatch and Jonathan D. Moreno, eds., "Consensus in Panels and Committees: Conceptual and Ethical Issues," *The Journal of Medicine and Philosophy* 16 (August 1991): 371-463.

made by Bruce Jennings in his article "Possibilities of Consensus: Toward Democratic Moral Discourse" served as our guide:

> Consensus in the strongest sense of the term happens only when it is seen as a common good to be created, and thus the creation of consensus becomes a special civic intention shared by the participants in the moral dialogue...
>
> In seeking to develop a common sense of what their shared problems are, members of a community also develop a sense of what it is they have in common. In doing this their identity as moral agents can be transformed; they can experience their own moral agency more in terms of those aspects of experience that unite them to other agents and fellow participants and less in terms of those experiences that differentiate them.[41]

Based on Jennings' proposal, the conceptual frame of the project is composed of two lines of research. A first one is related to conflict management. A central concern of the specialists in the field is to develop a better understanding of how the theoretical and practical knowledge of the discipline could help promote, among the disputants, a mutual discovery and a greater comprehension. The analysts have proposed communication strategies,[42] techniques based on the intervention of a third party[43] or strategies based on the intervention of specialized teams.[44] These proposals aim at helping participants discover and appreciate values, interests and concerns that lie behind the positions of the disputants. Many analysts consider the process of transformation by which individuals become able to understand others as essential to conflict resolution. While conflicts of values seemed to resist strategies of intervention, resistance

---

41. Bruce Jennings, "Possibilities of Consensus: Toward Democratic Moral Discourse," *The Journal of Medicine and Philosophy* 16 (August 1991): 461.

42. Anatol Rapoport, *Fights, Games and Debates* (Ann Arbor: University of Michican Press, 1974); Howard Raiffa, *The Art and Science of Negotiation* (Cambridge: Harvard University Press, 1982); Robert Axelrod, *The Evolution of Co-operation* (New York: Harper and Row, 1985); Roger Fisher and Scott Brown, *Getting Together* (Harmondsworth: Penguin, 1989).

43. Christopher Moore, *The Mediation Process* (San Francisco: Jossey-Bass, 1986); Kenneth Kressel and Associates, *Mediation Research* (San Francisco: Jossey-Bass, 1989).

44. Susan Carpenter and W. J. D. Kennedy, *Managing Public Disputes* (San Francisco: Jossey-Bass, 1988).

may be overcome, according to recent studies, when participants begin to change the way they see the others.[45]

The theme of the "common good" constitutes the second line of research. In bioethics, Daniel Callahan has especially promoted the idea of the common good. He and other thinkers who stress the same idea are criticized because they would not take pluralism seriously.[46] What the critique does not recognize is the possibility of different interpretations of the common good. In fact, the common good need not be considered a static reality, it can be interpreted as a dynamic one. The concept of recurrence schemes proposed by Bernard Lonergan allows for such an interpretation: its meaning is to understand the links between the different values that exist within an ethical conflict.[47] The Lonerganian approach helps the individuals involved in an ethical dispute understand that the interaction between the various levels of values is rooted in the recurrence scheme. If the theory of conflict resolution indicates the means and abilities needed to transform the disputants, the theory of the common good understood as a dynamic reality allows these individuals to understand how their values, interpreted as conflictual, are in fact linked.

By proposing a method of deliberation that relies on differences and their richness, we hope to help health care teams become more creative in their commitment to sick people and their loved ones. This approach seems indeed the most appropriate for favouring the covenant relation between patients and health care professionals. By discovering the implicit ethics of the diverse professionals and the tension that exists between their respective ethics, professionals will be helped to focus on a patient's narrative.

---

45. Daniel Druckman, "Value Differences and Conflict Resolution: Facilitation or Delinking?" *Journal of Conflict Resolution* 32 (September 1988): 489-510; Tetsuo Kondo, "Some Notes on Rational Behavior, Normative Behavior, Moral Behavior, and Cooperation," *Journal of Conflict Resolution* 34 (September 1990): 495-530.

46. Ron Hamel, "Books," *Bulletin of the Park Ridge Center* (May 1990): 34-37.

47. Bernard Lonergan, *Insight* (New York: Philosophical Library, 1958); Bernard Lonergan, *Method in Theology* (New York: Herder and Herder, 1972); Patrick Byrne, "Jane Jacobs and the Common Good," in *Ethic in the Making*, ed. Fred Lawrence (Atlanta: Scholars, 1989), 169-189.

PART 1

**IMPLICIT ETHICS OF PROFESSIONALS
IN THE FIELD OF PEDIATRIC CHRONIC CARE**

Introduction to Part 1

Jean-Marc Larouche
and Tim Flaherty

One of the overall objectives of this study is to investigate how professionals involved in long-term care units in pediatric chronic care experience value conflicts and make decisions on ethical issues.[1] Therefore, we are interested in professionals as *moral agents*. Are they experiencing these value conflicts and making their ethical decisions as *moral reproducers*, referring to explicit codes or institutional standards; as *moral interpreters* of codes and standards in light of values such as dignity; or as *moral creators,* with emphasis on shared responsibility and on recognition of the complexity of the situations and the uncertainty of ethical decisions?

---

1. As co-researcher in this project, I had the responsibility of the documentary analysis from which a typology of the "Implicit Ethics of Professionals in the Field of Pediatric Chronic Care" would be set. To achieve this goal, I first formed a research team with three graduate students, Tim Flaherty, Jean-Louis Munn and Jean-Eudes Charbonneau, who were respectively in charge of the nurse, the physician and the social worker sections.

    The first year of the project was devoted to the conceptual and methodological formation of the team and to the collection of the relevant literature. During the second year, the documentary analysis in the field of nursing was completed by Tim Flaherty, and in the fields of physician and social worker by Jean-Eudes Charbonneau and Tim Flaherty. These analyses were progressively criticized, revised and improved through the discussions within our specific research team and with other co-researchers and their assistants in the general research team meetings.

    In the third year, Tim Flaherty had the responsibility of writing, under my direction and supervision, a synthesis report. He was also in charge of making the database available in electronic format (see Appendix A). Two undergraduates, Nancy Lepage and Melissa Trono, continue to assist him in this task. This part of the study, therefore, is the result of an ongoing research process in which students played a key role in different phases of the project. I wish to thank all of them for their successful assistance and collaboration. As Tim Flaherty became my right-hand man in this project over the years, I want to thank him especially for his dedication and for the professional and intellectual probity of his work.—Jean-Marc Larouche

Before conducting an empirical research through observation of clinical teams engaged in ethical deliberation, we undertook a documentary analysis to establish a *typology of the implicit ethics* of the principal professionals involved in the field of pediatric chronic care: the nurse (chap. 2), the physician (chap. 3) and the social worker (chap. 4).[2] It is our understanding that what lie behind values and decisions of these professionals as moral agents are most often "implicit ethics," rather than what is contained in statements of explicit ethics.

In fact, before explicitly tackling problems of an ethical nature, discussing them and then marking a path for oneself and others to follow, each person carries an implicit ethic. This, more precisely, is what the French sociologist Pierre Bourdieu calls an *ethos*:

> a system of durable and transposable dispositions that integrates all past experiences functioning at each moment as a *matrix of perceptions, appreciations and actions*, and makes possible the accomplishment of infinitely differentiated tasks by both analogical transfers of schemes allowing the resolution of problems of the same form and ceaseless corrections to the results obtained, corrections that are dialectically produced by the results obtained.[3]

Here we are interested, therefore, in aspects of the professional identity of nurses, physicians and social workers, and we are concerned with identifying those "dispositions to act, think, perceive, and feel" pertaining to these professionals when they are confronted with ethical problems, as well as examining how their professional socialization forms their respective manner of relating to ethics and ethical work.

From the literature regarding these professionals, in accounts of the histories and professional socialization of the individual professions and in the recently written works of these professionals, particularly in their journals, we looked for indicators of the values, understandings and attitudes that inform their action. These indicators are not always explicitly labelled as a value or a goal of the profession but are seemingly present in the ongoing *ethos* of the profession. *The methodology is therefore inductive*

---

2. The choice of these professions is based on their visible and influential role in the management of pediatric chronic illness. It is recognized that other professionals are involved and that parents or guardians in particular play a major role. Their participation is the subject of future research. For our purposes, the child-patient and the child's family are considered in their reactions to the three principal professions.

3. Pierre Bourdieu, *Esquisse d'une théorie de la pratique* (Geneva: Droz, 1972), 178-179; our translation.

and synthetic.[4] It proceeds from indicators or suggestions of schemes of valuing or acting, and from these develops dimensions or characteristics of a portrait of the professional that we will construct. These portraits will help us project potential conflicts when they are placed beside portraits of other actors addressing ethical questions or issues. In addition, these portraits will provide a tool of analysis for the second objective of this project, the guide of deliberation.

The portraits rely on the methodological concept of *ideal type* proposed by Max Weber as a tool for sociological analysis. An "ideal type" is a *construct* to obtain

> success in revealing concrete cultural phenomena in their inter-dependence, their causal conditions and their significance... An ideal type is formed by the one-sided accentuation of one or more points of view and by the synthesis of a great many diffuse, discrete, more or less present and occasionally absent concrete individual phenomena, which are arranged according to those one-sidedly emphasized viewpoints into a unified analytical construct... This conceptual pattern brings together certain relationships and events of historical life into a complex, which is conceived as an internally consistent system.[5]

It is important to note again that the portraits are constructs, *des tableaux de pensée*. The construct of the "ideal type" (or types) for each professional group provides a touchstone for observing and understanding the professional ethos and assessing the actions of each of these players considering that ideal type. It provides a vehicle for understanding how they approach ethics and the decision-making process. The ideal type of a professional as moral agent does not exist in itself. It is a construct that allows us to show trends in thinking and acting through the emphasis of differences. In reality, persons are a mix of the types. We note also that in characterizing by using "ideal type" we are not evaluating the types or their value or effectiveness in the health care enterprise. We propose this as a tool of analysis. "Ideal type" is used in the logical sense and not an ethical sense that implies what ought to be.

We note also that while distinctions between these dimensions or characteristics of portrait may be more evident in the literature than in

---

4. For a detailed description of the process of constructing this model of analysis and the terms used, see Raymond Quivy and Luc Van Campenhoudt, *Manuel de recherche en sciences sociales* (Paris: Bordas, 1988), especially 99-143.

5. See Max Weber, "Objectivity in Social Sciences and Social Policy," in *The Methodology of the Social Sciences*, trans. and ed. Henry A. Finch and Edward A. Shils (New York: Free Press, 1949), 50-112, especially 90-92.

clinical practice, they clearly overlap in theory and in history. In addition, we note here that these dimensions are not static but have evolved and are evolving. This evolution is influenced from outside the profession in the general cultural and social situation, religion and gender. Other influences are more specific and intrinsic to each profession. These include the process of formation and curriculum, issues of expertise, skill and knowledge, and the institution of practice. These factors all inform the individual's and the group's self-perception and role as professionals and their perception of the roles of others involved in the health care system.

The literature search conducted shows that there is no single portrait for each profession. Several identifiable portraits are operative in each profession involved in pediatric chronic illness, some more explicit than others. In addition, it quickly became evident that resident in each profession's understanding of itself and its role are the roots of conflict. The professions often excluded the role or influence of others in their evaluation of their own expertise, primacy or capacity for decision making. This will be made more evident in the following pages. The value of undertaking the second objective of the project, "the elaboration, proposal and evaluation of a guide of deliberation to orient the decision making of health care teams in pediatric chronic illness," has become evident.

A chapter is devoted to each profession considered. Each begins with a sociohistorical sketch that includes an account of events, evolution of attitudes and practices that help to account for the emergence of the ideal types of each profession. The ideal types that emerge from the literature search of materials in the field of pediatric chronic illness are then noted, followed by a section on the implicit ethics of each of the ideal types and their manner of addressing four ethical themes: autonomy, location of care, economics and decision making. Each chapter concludes with brief statements on the stance or orientation of the profession as moral agent.

Chapter 2

The Nurse as Moral Agent

Jean-Marc Larouche
and Tim Flaherty

INTRODUCTION

This chapter considers the profession of nursing as it is exercised in the field of pediatric chronic illness. We begin with a general sociohistorical sketch from which we observe the emergence of indicators that form the dimensions of the "implicit ethics" of three ideal types of nurses. This is followed by an illustration of how each of the ideal types addresses the four ethical themes of concern in this study: autonomy, economics, location of care and decision making. The chapter concludes with a synthesis that presents the nurse as moral agent and with concluding statements. In order to provide the general situation and context of the professionals involved in health care, this chapter is more detailed and lengthy than those that follow on the physician and the social worker. The details provided here will not be repeated in subsequent chapters but their importance will become evident.

SOCIOHISTORICAL PERSPECTIVE: THE TENSION BETWEEN CARING AND EXPERTISE

To focus on the aspects of nursing history that are significant for this chapter, the following sketch will be presented by observing the tension between two poles that define nursing.[1] The first is nursing *care* and the second is nursing *skill or technical expertise*. The literature suggests these poles are recognized as central points of orientation in a discussion of nursing practice. From our observation of the interplay of these poles, we

---

1. For greater detail and further documentation, see T. J. Flaherty, "Nursing Ethics: The Transformation of an Ethical Field," Research Services, Saint Paul University, Ottawa, August 31, 1993.

note indicators that allow us to identify the dimensions of three portraits, or ideal types, of nurse practising in the field of pediatric chronic illness.

Nursing has its origins in the art of caring practised as part of family living.[2] It became organized under monastic communities and religious orders after the rise of the influence of Christianity in the fourth century. It largely functioned as part of the "hospitality" monasteries offered to pilgrims. The practice of the art of nursing gradually became recognized as a vocation with the religious or moral motivation of charity. Its practice extended beyond the family circle to include care for the infirm and the poor. In this vocational expression, nursing was essentially the work of women. Women were assigned the role of caregiver by virtue of an understanding of the natural order.[3] Because of the social order of the time, the assignation of care as a feminine virtue devalued it as a form of subservience and as secondary to masculine virtues associated with power, authority and control. The valuing of care as a religious virtue, particularly in the exercise of charity, made remuneration for nurses inappropriate. As with all aspects of religious and monastic life, the virtue of obedience was highly valued. The nurse offered the patient comfort and care while following the direction of the physician and those in authority.

This understanding of nursing and its attribute of care was largely unchallenged in any formal manner until the time of the Crimean War in the 1850s and the British military nurse Florence Nightingale. Nightingale insisted on the recognition of the cognitive as well as the moral aspects of nursing. She highlighted newly emerging nursing knowledge and capability to illustrate non-moral good.[4] Nurses were to promote health as a science and engage in disease prevention. The cognitive aspect of nursing was an addition to the moral aspects of care that featured sacrifice, charity and pity. This is a benchmark in the gradual transformation of nursing from *vocation* to *profession*.[5] It is significant to note here that although tremendous influence is credited to Nightingale for moving nursing forward as a profession, she maintained that nurses must be obedient to the physician, give self-sacrificing care to the patient, assist the physician in his task and grow in the knowledge of the

---

2. See especially Teresa A. Christy, "Historical Perspectives on Accountability," in *Current Perspectives in Nursing Education*, vol. 2, ed. Janet A. Williamson (St. Louis: C. V. Mosby, 1978), 1-7; and Winnifred Gustafson, "Motivational and Historical Aspects of Care and Nursing," in *Care: The Essence of Nursing and Health*, ed. Madeleine M. Leininger (Detroit: Wayne State University Press, 1988), 61-75.

3. Gustafson, "Motivational and Historical Aspects of Care and Nursing," 69.

4. Ibid., 67.

5. For a detailed discussion of this phenomenon, see André Petitat, *Les Infirmières: De la vocation à la profession* (Montreal: Boréal, 1989).

nursing role. Nightingale saved many lives through will and determination in the face of opposition from traditional physicians. She insisted on a level of organization and personal and environmental cleanliness that was formerly unheard of in health care. She did not, however, seem to advocate the same attitude of opposition in her subordinates. Although her work in the war and in establishing nursing schools after her return to England offered some level of legitimacy and of acceptance of women working outside the home, as well as a degree of independence from the male-dominated medical hierarchy, Nightingale continued to uphold the traditional nurse–physician relationship as valid.

In the early years of this century, care given by nurses was offered to the patient largely as presence and comfort. Nurses had little formal training and acquired their skills through a loosely organized apprenticeship. They functioned primarily as private duty nurses in a patient's home, followed the physician's orders and showed their skill in tact and "the little things" that exemplified their dedication to the sick.[6] Working alone, they were largely self-directed and extended their care to the family of the sick individual.

Lacking the financial backing that allowed for the existence of independent and university medical schools to educate physicians, training for nurses was picked up by hospitals, which established schools as a source of cheap labour. The lack of autonomy in nursing training moved it away from Nightingale's focus on improved education, which would have allowed nurses to make responsible decisions in clinical settings. Canada followed international trends in nursing education. The first hospital diploma nursing school in Canada was established in St. Catharines in 1874.[7] Courses in simple anatomy, physiology, sanitary science, hygiene and practical matters of observation to help the physician were taught to students of "good character and Christian motivation." A school opened in Montreal in 1880, and another opened in Toronto in 1881.

During the Depression the situation changed again, this time due to economic pressures. Hospitals found it cheaper to employ graduate nurses than large numbers of students. This marked the practical end of "private duty" in individuals' homes. As the world pulled out of the Depression, World War II pulled the nurses out of the hospitals, where they were again replaced by students, who functioned along with nurses' aides to fill the

6. Sarah E. Dock, "The Relation of the Nurse to the Doctor and the Doctor to the Nurse," *American Journal of Nursing* 17 (1917): 395.

7. Janet Ross Kerr, "The Origins of Nursing Education in Canada: An Overview of the Emergence and Growth of Diploma Programs," in *Canadian Nursing: Issues and Perspectives*, 2nd ed., ed. Janet Ross Kerr and Jannetta MacPhail (Toronto: Mosby Year Book, 1991), 232.

vacuum.[8] Nurses returned from the war with an experience of having new responsibilities thrust upon them in the conflict and having acquitted themselves well. They returned to the hospitals, where they began to acquire new technical and medical skills. In part, this expanding scope of nursing resulted from marked changes in medical practice and the treatment of disease. For example, when diseases such as typhoid, influenza or other epidemics were no longer a threat, the need for the private duty nurses they had occasioned disappeared and opened opportunities for new areas of nursing practice.

With the return of nurses to the hospital, students were directed to spend more time in studies. Graduate nurses also advanced their knowledge in areas such as pathology, physiology and anatomy. Their expanding scope of influence, however, was not limited to the medical. In their return to the hospital, nurses began to enter the bureaucracy as participants in the hierarchical structure.[9] They began to work *with* others. This consequently changed the work *of* others, such as physicians and patients, and their relationships with other nurses. Still under the directions of physicians, whose orders they were to carry out, nurses supervised and directed other workers such as housekeeping and dietary staff. Nursing skills, along with medical skills, were now augmented by time management skills with their economic component.

It is significant to note here that the situation of the nurse in the hierarchical structure of the hospital was complex. As an employee of the institution, she was responsible to the administration for her performance. Simultaneously, the nurse was responsible for carrying out the orders of the physicians. Physicians were not always institutional employees and existed to some degree outside the institutional structure, while exerting great influence on the manner in which it conducted its affairs. As nurses entered the hospital bureaucracy, they also entered a new era in education. Nursing education expanded and advanced. While nursing had entered the university in 1919 in British Columbia, there had not been great progress on this front. In the fifties and sixties, private nursing schools began to appear as did possibilities for graduate research and education. Along with the bureaucratization of nursing, the increasing emphasis on the advances in medical science and technology began the shift from the nursing model of "care" to the medical model of "cure." Nursing began to change radically with this movement.

---

8. Marlene Kramer, "Educational Preparation for Nurse Roles," in *Current Perspectives in Nursing Education*, vol. 1, ed. Janet A. Williamson (St. Louis: C. V. Mosby, 1976), 95-118.

9. Kramer, "Educational Preparation for Nurse Roles," 96.

It is acknowledged by most authors in the field of nursing and nursing philosophy that technology has seriously challenged nursing's ability to care.[10] The influence of the "medical model" of cure has continued today. While many people enter nursing because of a desire to care for people and see caring as an inherent value in nursing, there remains pressure to put technology first in nursing practice. This poses an inherent problem within nursing. Care was something of a casualty in the technological shift to the medical model of health care. However, the shift was not the only factor. During their professional socialization, nurses were also confronted with the paradox of the ideal of caring and the warning that, as professionals, they should keep their distance and not get "too involved."[11]

In recent years, there have been an increasing number of books and articles written by nurses and nurse educators who recognize that there has been a loss of and appreciation of care as a central nursing value. Kramer offers the following appraisal of the situation:

> Today, technological skills play an enormous part in how the nurse directly helps the physician and the patient. Furthermore, because the increase in technological knowledge seems to have commonly decreased the intimate, personal relationship once existing between patient and physician, the nurse increasingly is donning the supportive role the physician once held. Where once the nurse's main emphasis was to care for patients directly, it is now often to see that they are cared for, or to "nurse" the desk, the organization or the computer.[12]

In the face of this reality, nurses are calling for a clearer expression of the philosophy of care in nursing to "direct nurses to the purpose of nursing interventions, remind staff of their commitment to each individual, and delineate boundaries with other disciplines, but more importantly it will unite nurses in their common-stated beliefs and values."[13] The care of which Leininger speaks as "the essence and the central, unifying, and dominant domain to characterize nursing"[14] is not essentially what

---

10. See authors such as Albarran, Gaut and Bevis, who deal extensively with the issue.

11. See Carol Leppanen Montgomery, "The Spiritual Connection: Nurses' Perceptions of the Experience of Caring," in *The Presence of Caring in Nursing*, ed. Delores A. Gaut (New York: National League for Nursing, 1992), 39.

12. Kramer, "Educational Preparation for Nurse Roles," 99.

13. J. W. Albarran, "Advocacy in Critical Care Nursing: An Evaluation of the Implications for Nurses and the Future," *Intensive and Critical Care Nursing* 8 (1992): 51.

14. Madeleine Leininger, "Care: The Essence of Nursing and Health," in *Care: The Essence of Nursing and Health*, ed. Madeleine Leininger (Detroit: Wayne State University Press, 1988), 3.

modern nursing speaks of as "quality of care" with its attendant implications of technological competence, but rather the personal, individual care offered in human presence. Nursing care contrasts sharply with medical cure, which is "more dramatic, male, technological and physical."[15] Care is assistive, supportive or facilitative. These expressions of the understanding of the place of care in nursing reflect what is to be found in the current literature. It reflects the exercise of the technical in the context of the personal.

We turn now to a consideration of the other pole that orients nursing practice, that of nursing skill. In the foregoing section on the virtue of care, much historical data was presented to create a context for the discussion. The same data is pertinent to the discussion of skill or expertise. For our brief discussion here, the two major points of interest are the content of skill and the focus of that skill.

One hundred years ago, tasks such as the taking of a patient's temperature were not thought of as falling within the realm of nursing care. This was part of diagnosis and treatment, which were the physician's responsibility. Today, nurse-practitioners diagnose, treat and even perform minor surgery with medical supervision. This constitutes a great change in the content of skill.

The process of this change in nursing skill and the scope of nursing competence is partly due to the social changes previously outlined, but also due to the advances in the sciences. Nursing began in prescience and evolved toward participation in the scientific enterprise.[16] Elimination of some diseases and advances in the diagnosis and treatment of others changed nursing and medicine. When it was perceived as possible, active treatment was added to comfort and compassion. Nurses began by following the directions of the physician and now entered health care exercising initiative and a degree of autonomy.

The knowledge acquired by nurses followed scientific discovery. Studies in pathology, anatomy and biology were joined by pharmacology and the behavioural sciences. Tact was never abandoned but it soon lost its place to more scientific ventures. As the field of medicine advanced, so did nursing. By joining in the medical model of "cure," nursing reflected general changes in medicine. Specialization by physicians was reflected in specialization of nurses and in similar areas—from neonatology to gerontology there are nursing specialities. In each of these areas, at whatever stage in its history, nurses placed upon themselves an

15. Leininger, "Care: The Essence of Nursing and Health," 4.

16. Martha E. Rogers, "Emerging Patterns in Nursing Education," in *Current Perspectives in Nursing Education*, vol. 2, ed. Janet A. Williamson (St. Louis: C. V. Mosby, 1978), 1.

expectation of excellence. With the technological revolution of the 1960s, nursing devoted itself to technology. With the appropriation of a health promotion role and the development of public health nursing, the nurse as educator emerged in a more formal way. Attributes not traditionally associated with those of nursing became important skills for the nurse. Communication, personnel and economic management are but three.

THREE PROFESSIONAL IDEAL TYPES OF THE NURSE

From the literature discussing the sociohistorical context of nursing, there emerge two predominant metaphors that evoke two "ideal types," or portraits, of nurses. The older of these is the "military metaphor," the more recent is the "advocacy metaphor."[17] For our purpose here, we label the nurse who practises in accord with the military metaphor as "the Manager" and label the other type of nurse as "the Advocate." Nurses educated and socialized in one or another of these above models are evidenced as practising in the field of pediatric chronic illness today. The older of the metaphors, nursing as military effort, which gives us the Manager, is not as explicit as advocacy in recent literature. Yet the literature indicates that there are nurses who still hold and practice the values and the traditions of this approach to nursing today.[18] The notion of advocacy, either as a legal notion or as advocacy of self-determination of the patient, is the dominant metaphor in recent literature. There is, however, a third model, or metaphor, observed in the literature. It is not labelled in the literature as are the others because it appears as an emerging model. We label it here as "the Coordinator." After presenting the types, we then briefly examine some examples of the literature that deal with cases and situations in which nurses find themselves. In doing so, we can uncover further dimensions to help sketch our portraits.

---

17. Gerald R. Winslow, "From Loyalty to Advocacy: A New Metaphor for Nursing," *Hastings Center Report* 14 (June 1984): 33. Winslow proposes that changes in metaphor are the most significant attestation to changes in the self-perception of nurses. His perspective is applicable to the other professions under consideration. Winslow sees the metaphors interacting with rules of conduct and principles to support or produce change.

18. For an example of this approach to nursing, see Lisa H. Newton, "In Defence of the Traditional Nurse," *Nursing Outlook* 29 (June 1981): 348-354.

The Manager

The literature presents nursing as military effort and nursing as advocacy of patients' rights.[19] Sarah Dock wrote in 1917 that the nurse was expected to be an intelligent machine that functioned, without question, in loyal obedience to the physician.[20] Working under the military metaphor also required the nurse to be technically competent in the limited scope allowed to her as she lived her vocation to care for the sick. Loyalty demanded faithful, self-sacrificing care of patients but also maintenance of confidence in the health care system by refusal to criticize her school, hospital, fellow nurses and, particularly, the physician. Nurses were to be prepared in the war against disease and sickness to endure hardships, danger, toil and discipline in their uniformed standing of duty to attain a professional manner—a central goal of nursing. Nursing was largely associated with female role-related characteristics and stereotyping— feminine, motherly, submissive and passive—in the face of physicians— masculine, paternal and dominant. This suited the military metaphor. Through the social and economic changes of this century, the nurse as military assistant has evolved to what we call the Manager, as this nurse implements the doctor's orders and hospital policy. The Manager seems to be an apt label for this ideal type because of the institutional orientation of this type's pattern of work. We reiterate here that the ideal type does not exist in itself in reality. Each person is a combination of types. Nor do we intend an evaluation of the types in our labelling. For example, to say that the orientation of a type is "institutional" is not to suggest that this is at the expense of the patient or the family. It states, rather, that this type follows the institutional practices and prescriptions as a norm. These practices in a health care setting are for the treatment and the benefit of the sick individual.

The Advocate

The second dominant metaphor in the literature is that of nursing as advocacy. Its appearance followed some events external to nursing and accompanied others from within it. Legal decisions called into question the traditional relationship of nurse and physician. There were significant changes in the educational and socio-economic distances between these two professions. Technological changes and advances in educational op- portunities for nurses allowed them to challenge the traditional power

---

19. See especially Winslow, "From Loyalty to Advocacy: A New Metaphor for Nursing," 32-40.

20. Dock, "The Relation of the Nurse to the Doctor and the Doctor to the Nurse," 394- 396.

structure in health care and its delivery. The events of the 1960s and 1970s gave rise to consumerism, the patients' rights movements and particularly the feminist movement. Each of these was to have a significant effect on the new metaphor of nursing as advocacy.

The language of advocacy was initially legal language and centred around protecting the rights of the patient, particularly the right to make decisions in health care. Nursing loyalty shifted to the patient, to protect against poor care or infringement of any rights by the institution or other health care workers. In emphasizing patient autonomy, nurses were initially concerned with providing information and obtaining fully informed consent from patients, without the nurse entering the decision-making process at all.

More recently, Sally Gadow and others have promoted an understanding of an "existential advocacy" as the philosophical foundation of nursing care.[21] The role of the nurse is one of offering assistance to the patient in determining and clarifying his or her own values and then making decisions based on those values. This promotion of self-determination of the patient is sharply contrasted with paternalism or patients' rights advocacy, which is largely a legal notion.

The Coordinator

As noted above, this is an emerging metaphor. Joy Henson Penticuff has extensively considered Gadow's work on existential advocacy and proposes a covenant model based on a promise to care.[22] The focus of this model is promotion of the child's determining self. This promise to care has as its component parts technical expertise, the giving of comfort, giving information and explanations to the child and family, inclusion of child and family in decision making, and the assurance the child and family will not be abandoned in the execution of the decision reached.

The literature on practical cases and situations yields the following examples: (1) The family of a severely disabled child feels powerless in the face of professionals who have neglected the family's autonomy by not informing them of their role in decision making.[23] The nurse undertakes to provide the parents with information that allows them to clarify

---

21. Sally Gadow, "Existential Advocacy: Philosophical Foundations of Nursing," in *Nursing: Images and Ideals: Opening Dialogue with the Humanities*, ed. S. Spicker and S. Gadow (New York: Springer, 1980).

22. Joy Henson Penticuff, "Ethics in Pediatric Nursing: Advocacy and the Child's Determining Self," *Issues in Comprehensive Pediatric Nursing* 13 (1990): 221-229.

23. Katherine M. Moore and René A. Day, "Child Care and Family Autonomy: Empowerment Through a Model for Ethical Decision Making," *Humane Medicine* 9, no. 2 (April 1993): 131-140.

their goals for their child's care and to make autonomous decisions. The result of the family's involvement is the feeling their child, rather than just his physical problems, is being treated. (2) In the case of disagreement between parents and the health care team as to the best course of treatment for a child, the nurse is proposed as the best professional to facilitate balanced judgment.[24] This is based on a perceived skill to seek information, balance perspectives, provide guidance, assess parental understanding and information needs, and facilitate communication, all in a way that avoids paternalism at all costs. The nurse's expressed goal in this situation is to assure protection of the child's needs, rights and comfort and those of the parents. (3) In the case where consideration is given to withdrawing/withholding treatment, nurses hold that life is precious and that the sanctity of life doctrine is the basis for nursing practice.[25] Nurses hold that the nurse–patient relationship is a covenant based on trust. (4) In neo-natal intensive care units (NICUs), the nurse's role is to aid parents in making life decisions for their child.[26] They do so in patient protection and the promotion of health and decision making in others. The nurse also helps the families in dealing with their reactions to their child and explains the treatment options. As a minister for health services, nurses must also recognize that ethical principles are directly related to the legal aspects of health care. (5) In the treatment of a child with cystic fibrosis, the nurse has an obligation to the family, for the sake of the child, to be attentive to changing patterns of interaction that may signal the onset of crisis or dysfunction.[27] Early intervention can avoid a crisis such as the hospitalization of the child for family respite, when such hospitalization is not warranted. (6) In making difficult decisions, especially those involving withdrawal/withholding of treatment, the health care professional must share the decision making with the family.[28] Nurses need to clarify the point where medicine meets human values.

In these examples, the nurse is seen to exercise the promise to care in compassion for the child and the family, in education and values clarification and in accompanying the child and family in decision making. These

---

24. Nancy K. Case, "Substituted Judgment in the Pediatric Health Care Setting," *Issues in Comprehensive Pediatric Nursing* 11 (1988): 303-312.

25. Susan J. Lagaipa, "Suffer the Little Children: The Ancient Practice of Infanticide as a Modern Moral Dilemma," *Issues in Comprehensive Pediatric Nursing* 13 (1990): 241-251.

26. Dixie L. Harms and James Giordano, "Ethical Issues in High Risk Infant Care," *Issues in Comprehensive Pediatric Nursing* 13 (1990): 1-14.

27. Susan Reed, "Potential for Alterations in Family Process: When a Family Has a Child with Cystic Fibrosis," *Issues in Comprehensive Pediatric Nursing* 13 (1990): 15-23.

28. Grant Gillet, "The Ethical Challenge of Sick Children," *Pediatrician* 17 (1990): 59-62.

actions and activities come from within the profession and are not imposed by the health care system. They suggest the particular ethos of the nurse that generates the explicit ethics of the profession. They are legitimized by the promise to care and the acceptance of the role of advocate in which nurses exercise a responsibility to assure the self-determination of the patient or, for a child, the potential determining self. There is also mention of obligation and duty to prevent alienation of the patient and family and assure their autonomy. The inclusion of legal considerations is something of a paradox in our portrait. Its centre is not client protection particularly, but also the protection of the nurse. Legal considerations, along with the reference to the doctrine of the sanctity of life, reflect aspects of the military metaphor. The other dimensions mentioned refer us to the advocacy metaphor. In developing our constructs of the ideal type, incidents of such paradox are not unusual. We do not ignore them. Rather, we go back to the understanding of Weber, which reminds us that this analytic construct accentuates some characteristics and synthesizes others to reveal concrete cultural phenomena.[29]

In summary, while we see indicators that there are evident dimensions of the two dominant metaphors in the literature covered to this point, there also appears to be a third model emerging. There are indicators of a change in self-perception, a change in the ethos within nursing. This third model is not military in its loyalty and obedience to the physician. It is not advocacy in terms of rights protection. It is more than advocacy of individual self-determination for the patient. It appears to be a third model perhaps rising out of the paradoxes found in the combinations of the first two. This emerging model sees the nurse aligned with neither the physician nor the patient, but somewhere in the centre as a facilitator of communication and ethical delivery of health care. Although an appropriate label for this nurse will await this metaphor's further development, for our purpose here it will be called "the Coordinator."

NURSES AND THEIR IMPLICIT ETHICS

We recall here once again that our methodology is *inductive and a work of synthesis*. From indicators in the literature, we had pieced together dimensions to form three professionals' ideal types of nurses. From the same literature we now move to an exploration of how these ideal types approach ethical issues in practice. That is to say, what values, attitudes and approaches form the implicit ethics that guide the decision making of each type.

---

29. Weber, "Objectivity in Social Sciences and Social Policy," 50-112.

As already noted, an earlier project of the Centre for Techno-Ethics, "Technology and Chronic Illness," identified four ethical issues seen to be central to any discussion of this question. They are autonomy, location of care, economics and decision making. This section of the chapter on the involvement of the nurse in the field of pediatric chronic illness offers examples or indicators of how each of the three nursing portraits address these issues. More examples can be found in this project's database. Presenting indicators of each portrait's manner of addressing an ethical issue will make the distinctions between them more explicit and make comparison possible within the professions.

The Manager

Autonomy

This approach to nursing views patient autonomy through the eyes of structure and organization that serve the medical needs of the child-patient. Language such as that used by Harms and Giordano employs words such as advocacy but has as an underlying basis, a deontology that requires beneficence (doing good and no harm) carry more weight than parental concerns when there is disagreement with health care professionals. When there is disagreement, it is the nurse's responsibility to help parents understand "treatment plans ordered by physicians." Furthermore, the "role of the nurse as a minister for health services and emotional physical well-being is built on the adherence to stringent ethical principles that are directly related to the legal aspects of medical care."[30]

A similar approach is also found in Murphy. There is primacy given to traditional deontological principles. For example, beneficence is defined as doing good; the good is determined by the nurse as is harm.[31] The language is heavily legal in terms of duty.

Location of Care

Developments in medical care and health management allow children who in the past would have died of their illnesses to survive. In many cases of chronic illness these children are no longer confined to institutions. It is now recognized by much of the health care system that hospitals and long-term care facilities are not the most appropriate place for all children to cope with chronic illness, nor are they always necessary. This movement

---

30. Harms and Giordano, "Ethical Issues in High Risk Infant Care," 12.

31. Jane M. Murphy and Nancy E. Famolare, "Caring for Pediatric Patients with HIV: Personal Concerns and Ethical Dilemmas," *Pediatric Nursing* 20, no. 2 (March 1994): 174.

in health care is responded to, in differing ways, by each of the three portraits of the nurse we are sketching.

In a discussion of pediatric chronic illness and the formation of the clinical nurse specialist for this practice, it is recognized that the positions available are in hospitals, schools and clinics, rehabilitation centres, and through public health offices.[32] While behavioural sciences are acknowledged, the emphasis is on the technology of the medical sciences. The focus is on the nurse specialists as managers for chronically ill children from hospital admissions and treatment, to ongoing care in community or institutions through transfers to varied institutions. There is no mention made of any type of consultation or discussion with family or child-patient. Haas writes of former days when the participation of parents was not solicited, as professionals were in charge of children.[33] The Barnes article appears to suggest the former days are not all gone. In dealing with the issue of location of care there are no significant indicators that distinguish a specific attitude on the part of this nurse.

Economics

The question of resources in terms of personnel, material and the health care dollar is present in almost any discussion today in the field of health care. Pediatric care is no exception. Resources are finite or perhaps even diminishing in terms of available dollars, while possibilities are expanding exponentially in terms of medical and technological advances. Each portrait sketched here presents a slightly different approach to balancing the two situations. It is interesting to note that in the nursing literature there was not a great deal of emphasis given to the economic issues perhaps because of a sense that this is beyond the control of the clinical nurse.

In recognizing the vast sums of money expended in NICUs on compromised neonates, the nurse inspired by the military metaphor asks if the money might better be spent elsewhere for greater beneficence. The response is an approach that understands utilitarianism while acknowledging they are bound to "a deontological set of ethics ... [and] are left with only the responsibility of formulating sound ethical, legal, and professional guidelines for action."[34]

---

32. Corrinne M. Barnes, "Training Nurses to Care for Chronically Ill Children," in *Issues in the Care of Children with Chronic Illness: A Sourcebook on Problems, Services, and Policies*, ed. Nicholas Hobbs and James M. Perrin (San Francisco: Jossey-Bass, 1985), 501-504.

33. Dianne L. Haas, Herman B. Gray and Beverly McConnell, "Parent/Professional Partnerships in Caring for Children with Special Health Care Needs," *Issues in Comprehensive Pediatric Nursing* 15, no. 1 (1992): 40.

34. See Harms and Giordano, "Ethical Issues in High Risk Infant Care," 10.

Decision Making

Decision making is the central ethical issue of our study. Its component parts are aspects of the other ethical issues covered, as well as personal and professional perspectives that have their roots in a sociohistorical context. For our purpose here, an outline of the general thrust or orientations that each portrait brings to decision making will be provided.

The approach to decision making here is one that requires a consideration of legal and ethical consequences of actions as well as of professional codes. "The role of the nurse as a minister for health services and emotional and physical well-being is built on the adherence to stringent ethical principles that are directly related to the legal aspects of medical care."[35] A discussion is recommended for those involved in making life-or-death decisions. In cases where there is ongoing care for a child, a nurse as manager of care will, with the health care team, oversee health care delivery. Such a portrait is characterized by a self-perception of their role as professional, educator, parent or follower and will deliver what is morally expected of them.[36]

The Advocate

Autonomy

Bartholome urges that nurses be recognized as the primary care providers to hospitalized children and infants and as the ones who are most intimately involved with their care and the decisions that affect it.[37] Health care professionals, including nurses and perhaps especially nurses, have a "fiduciary contract with the child-patient" and "by virtue of their social roles and relationships with their child-patients have legal and ethical duties and obligations which exist independently of any parental wishes, desires, and/or 'consentings.'"[38] This extends to situations where the nurse may step in and replace parents in case management if they are temporarily not up to the task.[39] Harms echoes this understanding when stating that

---

35. Ibid., 12.

36. Sigrid Fry-Revere, "A Bioethics Consultant's Thoughts on Caring for Pediatric Patients with HIV," *Pediatric Nursing* 20, no. 2 (March 1993): 177-180.

37. William G. Bartholome, "Withholding/Withdrawing Life-Sustaining Treatment," in *Contemporary Issues in Paediatric Ethics*, ed. Michael M. Burgess and Brian E. Woodrow (Lewiston, N.Y.: Edwin Mellen Press, 1991), 37.

38. Bartholome, "Withholding/Withdrawing Life-Sustaining Treatment," 23.

while autonomy and parental authority are closely related, it may become the nurse's responsibility to aid in life decisions concerning the infant.[40]

Autonomy respects the right of non-interference and the freedom and dignity of the individual. Nurses are in a "unique position to protect against harm, as well as avoid harm as they provide care."[41] This is a position of protector of the patient from others in the health care system who may cause harm "by failure to discharge moral, social, or legal duties to care for or act reasonably toward others."[42]

Location of Care

The nurse who practises as advocate is present in a variety of settings. Haas lists the following locations of care and type of practice:

> They practice in a variety of settings, such as hospitals, homes, clinics, schools, extended care facilities, public health agencies, physicians' offices, and independent groups of individual practices. They act as direct care providers, educators, researchers, managers, and clinical specialists. Because of the variety of settings and roles and the magnitude in numbers, the ability of pediatric nurses to impact on the lives of children with special health care needs and their families is significant.[43]

Hymovich notes that in these settings it has been suggested that advocacy be the primary responsibility of nurses working in them. An important aspect of this advocacy role is "helping children and families understand and manipulate the systems providing care to them."[44] The thrust of advocacy is to see the child cared for in the setting best suited to them. The patient and family interpret what is "best."

39. Sandra Graham McClowry, "Pediatric Nursing Psychosocial Care: A Vision Beyond Hospitalization," *Pediatric Nursing*, 19, no. 2 (March 1993): 148.

40. Harms and Giordano, "Ethical Issues in High Risk Infant Care," 5.

41. Murphy and Famolare, "Caring for Pediatric Patients with HIV," 174.

42. Ibid., 174.

43. Haas, Gray and McConnell, "Parent/Professional Partnerships in Caring for Children with Special Health Care Needs," 42.

44. Debra P. Hymovich, "Nursing Services," in *Issues in the Care of Children with Chronic Illness: A Sourcebook on Problems, Services, and Policies*, ed. Nicholas Hobbs and James M. Perrin (San Francisco: Jossey-Bass, 1985), 483.

Economics

A note of distinction is raised in this portrait. While bound by the principle of fairness that compels equitable distribution of resources, decisions about treatment are examined according to their benefit to the patient and when resources are limited marginal benefit requires fiscally responsible allocation. This point of view separates the individual patient from societal decisions about allocation of resources.[45]

Decision Making

The primary approach of the nurse in this portrait includes "a commitment to 'protect' patients and to promote health and decision making in others. The nurse's primary responsibility is to the patient."[46] This nurse may assist a parent in the case management for a child or advocate for families with other health care professionals. Such nurses will give what is morally expected and more in difficult situations.

The Coordinator

Autonomy

This portrait incorporates aspects of the military and advocacy metaphors and adds a particular emphasis. In considering technology-dependent children and those who are indefinitely hospitalized, the consumption of health care resources is discussed, as is "the cost of unmet developmental, intellectual, emotional, and psychosocial needs[, which] is immeasurable to the individual child, the family, and ultimately to society."[47] A system of medical foster homes is proposed as a solution where nurses function as coordinators of an interdisciplinary team that collaborates with community and government agencies. The scope of the nurses' activity is to compensate for lack of parental and societal support by planning and coordination of care with a team, communicating plans and goals, providing a model of parenting behaviour, advocating for the child in all situations and "acknowledging value and worth to the child."[48]

---

45. C. Hylton Rushton et al., "End of Life Care for Infants with AIDS: Ethical and Legal Issues," *Pediatric Nursing* 19, no. 1 (January 1993): 82.

46. Harms and Giordano, "Ethical Issues in High Risk Infant Care," 12.

47. LaCrecia J. Britton and Janet D. Johnston, "Dependent on Technology: A Child Grows Up Hospitalized," *Pediatric Nursing* 19, no. 6 (November 1993): 584.

48. Britton and Johnston, "Dependent on Technology," 584.

The specific strengths of this nurse "include: (a) flexibility, (b) communication, and (c) collaboration."[49] These strengths can be employed in integrating medical, social and educational services for children and their families. While this may begin in a hospital, it extends beyond the institution into the community in whatever structures are appropriate for the child. The issues to be addressed include overcoming barriers, nurse-to-nurse referrals, collaboration with other disciplines to provide family-centred care and determining roles in care with parents, providers and professionals. There is a strong caution that nurses or other professionals are not to take on a parent's role and that parents are recognized as the primary providers of care. Pediatric nurses are aware of their ability to deliberately plan the evolution and development of their specialty through ongoing evaluation of the health care system for children with chronic illness and the role of nurses in their care.

Location of Care

This model, or ideal type, suggested by the metaphor is distinguishable from the preceding two in its inclusiveness of much of their direction, and provides some unique features. It is these distinguishing features that will be noted here and in following sections of this chapter. Authors often mention two in particular: collaboration and flexibility.[50] The principal purpose of these features is to effect family-centred care that recognizes the distinctiveness and unique needs of each patient and family. Parents are the primary caretakers of their children and can function well if they are given information and support. Parents are an integral part of the health care team and are thus accountable for their participation.

The Coordinator recognizes that the issues in decision making include the emotional dimension, and while he or she is perhaps in the best position to assess the understanding of patients and parents, there is a need to include others in the assessment. The inclusion of social workers is especially noted by Moore. Moore also notes that when a nurse is proactive and willing to take risks by bringing conflict out into the open, a process of resolution can then be followed.[51] The goal is education of parents in the process of making informed collaborative decisions.

Also significant in this metaphor is the work of Penticuff. As outlined in the preceding section, children are to be assisted in building a

---

49. Graham McClowry, "Pediatric Nursing Psychosocial Care," 147.

50. See especially Graham McClowry, "Pediatric Nursing Psychosocial Care," 146-148.

51. Moore and Day, "Child Care and Family Autonomy," 131-140.

sense of autonomy and self-determination. Understanding and assent is a component part of treatment regimes:

> for the pediatric patient, advocacy enables the ill child to achieve an integration of the lived body [through our comforting] and the object body [through our explanation of her condition and its treatment], without which the self-unity required for development of authentic self-determination will be impossible.[52]

Significant attention is directed to the family in this process as they are accepted as central to the comfort and the care of this child-patient. Should there be cause to intercede to protect the child, it is based on the consciously made promise to care. The intervention may be in comfort, education, clarification or in the form of relief from pain and other discomforts.

In engaging in a promise or a covenant to care, Penticuff accepts that the nurse is obliged on the practical level to find the means to overcome or compensate for barriers to care, either institutional or personal. The key here seems to be that the coordinator is committed to the relationship between the providers and the recipients of health care. Significant factors in promoting this relationship include nursing's ability to influence or change the medical protocol from a nursing point of view; the degree of acceptance of nursing as a critical element in the institution's function; the degree of skill, both technical and interpersonal, with which nurses function on the unit; and nursing administration's ability to influence or control hospital resources.

Economics

Very similar in approach to the other two portraits, the Coordinator would include specific safeguards to assure that technology is not used inappropriately and "to monitor how the balance of benefit and burden are interpreted."[53] This monitoring effort would also recognize the need to halt treatments when they are no longer beneficial. A further instance of monitoring is given in determining the most appropriate location of care for a child. A home setting is absolutely less costly and, with nurses providing education and support through coordination of services, it is often the best place for a child and the family.

---

52. Penticuff, "Ethics in Pediatric Nursing," 225.

53. Hylton Rushton et al., "End of Life Care for Infants with AIDS," 82.

Decision Making

This portrait suggests a nurse aware of duty and the need to protect a child from neglect, mistreatment or futile measures. A further key is the ability to listen to parents and actively seek their participation in the decision process. Through education, parents are helped to become respected participants in their child's care.[54] It is recognized as a process that "must consider: [a] the moral limits on parental choice; [b] the need to lighten the load of responsibility and guilt on parents...; [c] the wishes of the child; and [d] the need to be sensitive to the limits of one's responsibility and not play God in the lives of others."[55] This portrait suggests a nurse who may go beyond what is morally expected and engage in a praiseworthy effort.

Decisions made by this nurse recognize the uncertainty and the complexity of questions raised and their ethical import. In addressing this complex of possibilities, the nurse is counselled to be proactive in anticipation of treatment plans and to engage in evaluation, consultation and the establishing of support networks and procedural safeguards for child, family and caregivers.[56]

SYNTHESIS: THE NURSE AS MORAL AGENT

The Manager as Moral Reproducer

Our research revealed three main ideal types that are portraits of the nurse involved in pediatric chronic care. Once again, we note this is not an attempt to assess the effectiveness or the desirability of any one type. They are *constructs* that reflect sometimes one-sided emphasis for the purpose of showing trends in thinking and acting.

The first, the Manager, functioned as the label suggests, as a middle manager conscious of and guided by a duty toward the physician, the patient and the institution. Decision making is guided by this tripartite deontology and as such does not reflect a great deal of independent initiative. The explicit ethics of this nurse as moral agent are found in codes of conduct, standards of practice and institutional standards. There is a highly legal and deontological emphasis biased toward authority and the institution. Any indicators of an implicit ethics we found referred directly to

---

54. Nancy Butler Simon and Debbie Smith, "Living with Chronic Pediatric Liver Disease: The Parents' Experience," *Pediatric Nursing* 18, no. 5 (October 1992): 458.

55. Gillet, "The Ethical Challenge of Sick Children," 61.

56. Hylton Rushton et al., "End of Life Care for Infants with AIDS," 82, 83.

these explicit standards. The Manager as moral agent is not a moral creator but a *moral reproducer*. This is an example of what Kohlberg refers to as the conventional model of moral sophistication.[57] It refers to the conservative, to what is institutional and to what helps keep the institution as it is. Key influences are authority and utilitarianism.

The Advocate as Moral Interpreter

The Advocate approaches the nursing function with a sense of independence and even authority to make decisions or to act "on behalf of" those who need protection from others, including parents, or the health care system. In a refined version, the Advocate operates as an assistant to the child-patient and family to achieve the goals of self-determination. In this case, indicators demonstrate that in the implicit ethics of this type there is a shift from following codes to what "really counts" or what is really at stake—the values and the dignity of the person are what is to be promoted and protected. The Advocate is *moral interpreter*. Values are the standard for action or decision making. This is more a post-conventional morality that is value-centred because norms and codes have to be measured by the criteria of the dignity and the best interests of the child as a person, and not by the criteria of the institution. The problems raised here surround conflict of values and perceptions of dignity, where there is little consensus. For example, the Advocate defines autonomy in terms of values and rights, and not in terms of the institution, as the Manager might, but nurses may not agree among themselves or with others on the values inherent in autonomy.

The Coordinator as Moral Creator

The Coordinator approaches decision making from the perspective of the child/family within a health care system with numerous players, all of whom are involved in making the best decision possible in the particular situation. The Coordinator is a *moral creator*. Coordination brings together people, ideas and proposals. It sorts and develops them to arrive at the best decision possible in the given situation. According to the main trend of indicators, the implicit ethics of the Coordinator refer mainly to the notion of shared responsibility, which Guindon describes as another degree of the post-conventional stage. The decisions or actions undertaken

57. For a detailed understanding of the moral models discussed in the section of the report, see Lawrence Kohlberg, *The Philosophy of Moral Development: Moral Stages and the Idea of Justice* (San Francisco: Harper and Row, 1981); Kohlberg, *The Psychology of Moral Development: The Nature and Validity of Moral Stages* (San Francisco: Harper and Row, 1984); and André Guindon, *Moral Development, Ethics and Faith*, trans. Kenneth C. Russell (Ottawa: Novalis, 1992).

will be good if they are taken by a group of persons that includes the patient and parents. If the parents are absent or unavailable for the process for any reason, there is a felt responsibility to create an environment for the child to access some parent reference in the clinical team. This is a responsible reference to whom the child is able to respond and who will respond to the child.

CONCLUSION

Nurses engaged in the field of pediatric chronic illness bring resources to their practice that include an extensive collective experience of care for the sick in varied conditions and settings, well-founded skill in medical and technological practice and an ability to combine the two in a humane manner. Their vast number and consistent presence in the lives of children with chronic illness make their influence unparallelled in the health care enterprise. In not being generally associated with the power structures of health care, their ability to be present to individuals and families is less threatening and perhaps more welcome. This may lend the nurse to the role of intermediary or coordinator. This is most true of a nurse who as moral agent functions as a moral creator and is able to see the situation for what it is and act in a creative way for the benefit of all concerned, particularly the child.

However, nurses are limited in many ways. Their lack of association with power structures is in some ways an impediment to influence in those structures. Institutional dominance over nursing has led some to suggest that nurses are not free to be moral agents in situations where their moral obligations to the patient or family conflict with the interests of those who pay their salary.[58] It can be a choice between the patient and one's career. The context of nursing activity, and the social or institutional structure in which it is exercised, can affect nursing expression of values and commitment. There is the added difficulty of confusion or lack of precision among nurses themselves about their role and their influence. There are diverse opinions on the meaning of such functions as "advocacy" in health care. These limiting factors may mitigate against the nurse as moral agent having a full impact in the health care enterprise.

---

58. Roland R. Yarling and Beverly J. McElmurry, "The Moral Foundation of Nursing," *Advances in Nursing Science* 8, no. 2 (1986): 64.

SUMMARY CHART OF IDEAL TYPES AND IMPLICIT ETHICS OF THE NURSE IN THE FIELD OF PEDIATRIC CHRONIC ILLNESS

IDEAL TYPE AND IMPLICIT ETHICS: nurses as moral agents	ETHICAL ISSUES			
	AUTONOMY	LOCATION OF CARE	ECONOMICS	DECISION MAKING
THE MANAGER AS MORAL REPRODUCER— refers to explicit codes or institutional standards for decision making	Legal and deontological approach— autonomy defined by authority	Manager according to the best interests of the institution	Supports utilitarian approach	Deontological (consequentialist) by codes and standards not by principle
THE ADVOCATE AS MORAL INTERPRETER— interprets codes and standards in light of individual needs, values and dignity	Protector of the dignity of the individual	Advocate of the best interests of the child	Cost-benefit— focus in the best interests of the child	Patient-centred— refers to what is mutually expected
THE COORDINATOR AS MORAL CREATOR— emphasis on shared responsibility and recognition of complexity of situations and uncertainty of ethical decisions	Child family-centred— focus on self-determination	Collaborator with parental concerns	Beneficence toward the child	Shared responsibility— awareness of the complexity and uncertainty of ethical decisions

Chapter 3

The Physician as Moral Agent

Jean-Marc Larouche
and Tim Flaherty

INTRODUCTION

We present here a parallel to the chapter on nursing, keeping in mind that there will not be the repetition of much of the historical and social data that provide the context for our discussion. This chapter considers the physician and the exercise of this profession in the field of pediatric chronic illness. A brief historical sketch provides the background from which to observe the emergence of the indicators and the *implicit ethics* of three ideal types of physicians. This is followed by illustrations of how each of the ideal types addresses the ethical themes of autonomy, location of care, economics and decision making. A conclusion offers a synthesis of the information covered and discusses the physician as moral agent.

HISTORICAL PERSPECTIVE

A brief historical presentation is the background for a discussion of Veatch's four models of physicians and Kluge's work on models of physicians in a Canadian context. Using literature on pediatric chronic care, we note there are not clear examples of Veatch's models and we propose three ideal types of physicians drawn together from indicators found in the literature surveyed.

Medicine and its practice by particular individuals has a long and well agreed upon historical development. For this chapter we will provide a narrative account of this development and the sociohistorical events that accompanied it. It is intended as a sketch or background for the ideal types that are portraits of the physicians involved in pediatric chronic illness.[1]

---

1. Further information and details can be found in sources listed in the Bibliography, in the section corresponding to this chapter.

Early history provides evidence of a combination of healing arts and magic or religion in most primitive communal situations. The role of healer was taken seriously and often was held by someone in the position of priest, shaman or medicine man. Their function was to heal, make new discoveries and pass on the information from generation to generation within the priesthood to social cult that practised medicine. Outsiders were discouraged from seeking this knowledge. Egyptian medicine included diagnosis, treatment and suggestion for therapy, as well as prognosis, incantations, available prescriptions such as castor oil and tannic acid, and surgical directions. In ancient Israel, medical practice was a priestly function. Greek medicine was associated with the worship of Apollo and included prescriptions for diet, rest, exercise and magic. A prolific writer on medical matters was the Greek Hippocrates. Significant influence in the early practice of medicine following the fall of Rome is credited to the detail and precision of work in the Islamic empire.

The Middle Ages in Europe witnessed the great effect of Christianity upon medicine. The virtue of charity inspired hospitals. Theological dualism led to more concern with the soul than the body to the extent that disease was considered the result of spiritual defects and was, therefore, cured through spiritual means. This effectively halted the scientific enterprise for a time. The late Middle Ages saw the number of medical schools in Europe rise.

The Renaissance witnessed the transformation of human activity on all levels, especially the scientific and intellectual. Particular notice is given to the beginnings of accurate anatomy texts and humane surgery. Through the seventeenth to the nineteenth century, discoveries were made at an increasing rate in anatomy, pharmacology, surgery, microbiology, bacteriology and related diseases, anesthesia and the field of physical diagnosis.

Our own century has witnessed the most rapid advances in medicine that have coincided and taken advantage of the vast developments in related fields of science and technology. Antibiotics, vaccines, X-rays, nuclear medicine and diagnostic tools, and the development of new fields of research such as molecular genetics have revolutionized diagnosis, treatment and prevention of illness and disease. Our system of health care delivery has become increasingly complex.

In this century, health care began as the responsibility of the family physician, who diagnosed and treated illness by himself, employing unskilled help if any. Most physicians were general practitioners and those who were not were surgeons. Any specialists were to be found on the faculties of university medical schools. As progress in medical knowledge and technology advanced, so did the need for physicians to specialize. Today medicine recognizes 23 specialties such as internal medicine, pediatrics and surgery, each with its own subspecialties. Pediatrics deals with infants and children and more recently has extended care to adolescents. These groups are seen to have distinctive diseases and disease patterns. There are also distinctive subspecialties unique to pediatrics, including neonatal and perinatal care.

There is an increasing awareness by physicians that although science in general, and medicine in particular, continue to make advances, cure is not always possible. Attention is beginning to focus on the limitations of medicine and the results of medical interventions. Not many years ago, children who would not have survived because of their illnesses are alive and functioning in varying degrees in our society. There are new challenges presented by these lives. In other situations, medicine is learning to admit it can do little or nothing except give comfort and support. This is a great shift away from a "cure" model of medicine. It is not always accepted easily by certain physicians. For those who are comfortable with the shift, there is a growing awareness of the needs of patients beyond physical treatment and of other professions who are allied in the delivery of a spectrum of health care services. The physician need not stand alone.

This historical sketch allows us to suggest that there have been physicians who were priests, physicians who functioned as scientists, physicians who emphasized cure and some who collaborate with others in care as well as cure. Using this historical background, Robert Veatch[2] and others have identified at least four models or types of physicians that have emerged and practise medicine today. The first model is the Engineering Model. Here, because of technological advances in biology, the physician behaves in a scientific, factual and value-free manner. He is the applied scientist. The type of interaction with the patient is often limited to presentation of facts and carrying out the decision of the patient.

The second is the Priestly Model. This model describes the physician–patient relationship as religious, where the physician becomes a new priest. The roots of this association of medicine with religion and the physician with the priest are ancient. As the priest's practice and power relies traditionally on a sacred knowledge (*savoir sacré*), which is obscure to the laypeople, the physician's aura of power and his or her capacity to control also relies on a knowledge that remains obscure to the patient. There is also the capacity to transfer the scientific expertise of medicine to expertise in the moral area. This model is characterized by paternalism on the part of the physician who ascribes to the axiom of doing good and no harm. The physician's authority in this situation may be so

---

2.   Robert Veatch, "Models for Ethical Medicine in a Revolutionary Age," *Hastings Center Report* 2 (June 1972): 5-7.

dominant that the patient's freedom and dignity in making decisions for his or her own well-being is lost. This, then, affects the balance of other important moral themes in the ethical enterprise.

Veatch's third model is the Collegial Model. This model attempts to find a comfortable balance between fundamental values and obligations, where the physician and patient are colleagues who share a common goal of doing what is in the patient's best interest. The relationship is one of trust, confidence, dignity, respect, pleasant and harmonious interaction and, probably most important, an arena for equal value contributions. Given, however, the many ethnic, class, economic and value differences in our communities, Veatch proposes that it may be more realistic to focus on a more provisional model. He says this would encourage equality between the physician and the patient, without assuming collegiality.

The final model Veatch distinguishes is the Contractual Model. He intends that his notion of contract not be legalistic but symbolic in nature, as in the religious notion of "covenant." In this arrangement, the physician and the patient each have obligations, yet each is to receive certain benefits. Basic to this model are norms of truth-telling, promise-keeping and justice.

Veatch explains that it is only through the Contractual Model that true reciprocation of ethical authority and responsibility can be realized. This is because the moral abdication by the physician and the patient in the Engineering and Priestly Models respectively, and the false sense of equality in the Collegial Model, are all avoided. Instead, there is a real sharing of decision making. While the patient does not have to participate in every decision, he or she can rest assured that decisions by the physician and the medical community are being made based on his or her own values. This in turn demands that sufficient open communication and dialogue between both parties take place before medical decisions are made.

In support of the perspective taken by Veatch, Kluge writes of the Canadian context of physician practice. Basing his distinctions on the work of Veatch, Kluge outlines six models of the physician–patient relationship. Kluge's first four models are the Paternalistic or Priestly Model, the Agency or Engineering Model, the Collegial Model and the Contractual Model, and to these he adds the two models that follow.

The Friendship Model has similar characteristics to those of the Collegial and Priestly Models. However, in the friendship relationship, the physician's professional obligation to the patient not only stems from a legal obligation, but is also grounded in the personal relationship that the two share. Therefore, the patient's autonomy may be overridden to a certain degree, but always within a context of accountability, trust, good will and pursuing the patient's best interests.

The Fiduciary Model is one of trust. This model recognizes that the physician and the patient do not share the same status with respect to knowledge, control or authority, yet a level of balance is still sought between the two parties. The patient's autonomy is balanced against the physician's knowledge, expertise and own rights as both an individual and as a professional. The limits of this model, then, are wider than the Contractual Model, since it is advocating that the physician not be ethically required to provide care, when honouring that request would violate his or her own moral beliefs.

The preceding sections of this report outline the historical and practical models of the physician as described or characterized by models, particularly those of Veatch. These in brief are:

1. The Engineering Model or physician as applied scientist: Refers to one who uses knowledge and technology to execute that which is possible in the profession. This physician presents the facts to the patient and leaves the decision making to that patient.

2. The Priestly Model: The type of practice here is paternalistic—doing good and no harm in the best interests of the patient. This "best interest" is usually defined by the physician.

3. The Collegial Model: Here the physician and the layperson are equal colleagues who share common interests and concerns.

4. The Contractual Model: Here the physician and layperson are not equal but have mutual interests and share ethical authority and responsibility.

THREE PROFESSIONAL IDEAL TYPES OF THE PHYSICIAN

What first becomes evident in attempting to sketch portraits of the physicians involved in pediatric chronic care is that the literature surveyed does not provide discrete examples of the four models suggested by Veatch. However, certain aspects of each are evident. It is these aspects or dimensions that we will use to form the composites required for our purpose. The first type comprises dimensions that as a group are consistent with the models of the physician as engineer or scientist and the physician as priest; we will call this type "the Expert." Another type consists of dimensions that as a group are consistent with those of the Collegial or Contractual Model; we will call this type "the Collaborator." The last type involves dimensions that appear to be transitional between the two other groupings; we will label this type "the Team Leader."

The Expert

These physicians are focussed on the challenge presented by an illness and by the need to reaffirm their own "omnipotence" in the face of that challenge.[3] They do not necessarily perceive the outcome or broader implications of their interventions beyond the immediate situation. This group is composed of a large number of specialists who are called upon in a particular situation to address a crisis or need and then are gone from the scene. Current trends in medicine call for wide application of technology (i.e., equipment and procedures). These applications do not always include consideration of their wider effects upon the patient as a person.[4]

This physician bases medical decisions on the best interests of the patient considered individually.[5] Resource allocation questions consider the best interests of the patient and the interests of society, the physician and the hospital.[6] The moral principle of autonomy, codes of ethics and case studies of moral conflicts aid physicians in determining the course of action that respects the rights of patients. The good is decided by the physician.

While these physicians may recognize the need to expand their view beyond the biological need and good of the patient, they are not inclined to consider the expertise of those outside the profession. Physicians take for granted their benevolent intentions and ability to make the best judgments. They do not appreciate lawyers, rights advocates, moralists, legislators, economists and so forth interfering with their ability to deal with ethical dilemmas.[7] This approach to decision making sometimes has the effect of going day to day until a crisis forces change or a daily practice oriented around likes and dislikes and habit rather than ethical principles. Given either case, they take the interference of others badly.[8] This is a

---

3. Constance U. Battle, "Beyond the Nursery Door: The Obligation to Survivors of Technology," *Clinics in Perinatology* 14, no. 2 (June 1987): 418-419.

4. See Arlene McKenna Adler, "High Technology: Miracle or Malady for Patient Care," *Radiologic Technology* 61, no. 6 (July-August 1990): 478-481.

5. Charles Culver, *Ethics at the Bedside* (Hanover: University Press of New England, 1990).

6. Frederic Grunberg and John R. Williams, "Responsabilité morale des médecins en ce qui concerne la distribution des ressources en soins de santé," *Annals RCPSC* 21, no. 5 (July 1988): 312.

7. Leon R. Kass, "Ethical Dilemmas in the Care of the Ill," *Journal of the American Medical Association* 244, no. 16 (October 17, 1989): 1811-1816.

8. B. W. Neal, "Ethical Decision Making in Pediatric Practice: The Pediatrician and the Community," *Bulletin de l'Association Internationale de Pédiatrie* 4, no. 7 (July 1982): 6-10.

position of power that can cause any patient, especially a child, to see the physician as a rule maker within a reward/punishment system.[9]

The great number of technological advances causes these physicians to make decisions of greater depth and complexity. Authors in the field also note that increased liability, both civil and criminal, goes hand in hand with the more numerous decisions. The result is the practice of defensive medicine.[10] This is a form of legal jeopardy that occurs when legal liability replaces moral law.[11]

It is noted that pediatrics is "fertile ground" for paternalism when "arrogant physicians" do not share the decision-making processes but rather impose their views.[12] The experiences of parents with the Expert give us further insight into this type of individual's practice. Parents often feel frustrated in dealing with physicians as they experience exclusion from the decision-making process and difficulty in understanding the physicians' language and information, which is often too little and too vague. Parents feel that they are not regarded as competent by physicians.[13]

The central focus of the Expert is that of use of expertise and technology to provide the means to cure or alleviate illness to the greatest degree possible. Much of the commentary on the Expert is critical of this type's lack of holism in their approach to medicine, specifically in their manner of approaching illness in isolation from other aspects of the patient's life.

The Team Leader

There is a body of literature that, while critical of the Expert, points to directions for change. The central issue is a call for collaboration in health care decision making. There is often mention of a team approach of shared management for the benefit of the child, parents and team members. When the pediatrician takes charge or delegates this responsibility

9. Allan Lee Drash, "Juvenile Diabetes," in *Caring for Children with Chronic Illness: Issues and Strategies*, ed. Ruth E. K. Stein (New York: Springen Publishing Co., 1989), 155-182.

10. Odette Valabrègue-Wurzburger, "Legal Aspects of Ethics in Pediatrics," *Bulletin de l'Association Internationale de Pédiatrie* 4, no. 8 (1982): 5-10.

11. Culver, *Ethics at the Bedside.*

12. Alan R. Fleischman, "Ethical Views and Values," in *Caring for Children with Chronic Illness*, 92.

13. S. F. Diehl, K. A. Moffit and S. M. Wade, "Focus Group Interview with Parents of Children with Medically Complex Needs," Ph.D. diss., University of South Florida, 1991, 4-6.

to a specialist, fragmented care is avoided.[14] The collaboration and consultation do not, however, always include the family. It is often limited to communication between specialists and specialties.[15] Strayer notes that physicians are learning that shared responsibility can be positive (i.e., sharing between specialists), while many still maintain that specialists do not have time for communication with family and for case management.[16]

At the same time, there is a growing awareness that physicians are not technicians offering a service and that they recognize the need for discernment in providing care and development of a broader decision-making process.[17] Those educating physicians are encouraged to develop a self-awareness of their own power and ability to impose personal values on others because of their position. In entering the decision-making process with such an awareness of their role and their power, the possibility of reaching a truly common decision with a team is enhanced.[18]

It is interesting to note the language used when speaking of physicians on the health care team. While speaking of the physician's participation on a multidisciplinary team as "essential," the position that they occupy is a central one—that of "quarterback."[19] The same type of language is used in a recent article that focussed on communication of the pediatric neurosurgeon as a key factor in a child's recovery. "The pediatric neurosurgeon is the captain of the team which consists of other attendings, fellows, residents, medical students, physician assistants and nurse practitioners."[20] The physician may be on a team but remains "in charge." Awareness may have changed but practice does not always seem to have kept pace. In spite of calls for changes in the way physicians are educated

---

14. Jerome Fialkov, "Peregrination in the Problem Pediatric Patient: The Pediatric Munchhausen Syndrome?" *Clinical Pediatrics* 23, no. 10 (October 1984): 571-575.

15. See, for example, G. K. Fritz et al., "Pediatric and Psychiatric Collaboration in the Management of Childhood Asthma," *Clinical Pediatrics* 20, no. 12 (December 1981): 774, on the management of childhood asthma, where collaboration is between pediatric and psychiatric fields, and parents are not likely to be involved.

16. F. H. Strayer et al., "Physician Incentives for Shared Management of Childhood Cancer Patients," *Pediatrics* 67, no. 6 (June 1981): 836.

17. Claude Sureau, "Problèmes éthiques en période prénatale," *Bulletin de l'Association Internationale de Pédiatrie* 4, no. 7 (July 1982): 47-53.

18. Heleen Terborgh-Dupuis, "Training of Future Pediatricians in the Field of Ethics," in *Bulletin de l'Association Internationale de Pédiatrie* 4, no. 8 (October 1992): 11-13.

19. Chester D. Poremba, "Pediatrics and High Risk Youth: A Team Member's Perspective," *Developmental and Behavioral Pediatrics* 1, no. 1 (March 1980): 15-18.

20. Tania Shiminski-Maher, "Physician-Patient-Parent Communication Problems," *Pediatric Neurosurgery* 19 (1993): 104-108.

to improve the situation, a recent survey points out how little medical schools have changed in the last two decades.[21]

The Covenant Partner and Collaborator

Gillet and others recognize that there are special ethical issues present when one is dealing with children who are seriously ill. With all the skill and technology available and the challenge of difficult situations that arise, physicians need to engage in reflective judgments to avoid cruel and futile interventions and provide quality care and comfort. There is a definite need to recognize the limits of one's medical responsibility and not play God. Articles that advocate this approach emphasize that both parents and the child have wishes and need to be considered in the decision-making process.[22] Articles also note that there is a need to distinguish between the interests and the wishes of the parents and those of the child.[23] Here, it is necessary for the physician to be the advocate for the child, even opposing parental wishes. This includes issues surrounding interventions and withholding/withdrawing treatments.

This model recognizes that multidisciplinary collaboration is required to manage chronic illness in children. This collaboration is broad in its effort to normalize the life of chronically ill children and includes coordination of health care delivery, community-based health care and comprehensive health care planning.[24] The process of normalization includes consideration of cognitive, physical and social needs. In all these areas the parental role is central. It demands a broad degree of interdisciplinary (as distinct from multidisciplinary) cooperation that is medically, psychologically and rehab-oriented.[25] For the good of the child involved, the physician as sole health care director is not justified. Parents and especially nurses are acknowledged as integral.[26]

---

21. Anderson M. Brownell, "Medical Education in the United States and Canada Revisited," *Academic Medicine* 68, no. 6 (June 1993): 55-63.

22. See, for example, Lantos and Kohrman; Mallory and Stillwell; and Gillet.

23. See Bartholome; and Gillet.

24. Joan M. Patterson and Robert W. Blum, "A Conference on Culture and Chronic Illness in Childhood: Conference Summary," *Pediatrics* 91, no. 5 (May 1993): 1025-1030.

25. L. Singer et al., "Developmental Sequelae of Longterm Infant Tracheostomy," *Developmental Medicine and Child Neurology* 31 (1989): 224-230. Amelia Malfair, "Supporting the Child with Special Needs," *The Canadian Nurse* 88, no. 11 (December 1992): 18, distinguishes the multidisciplinary approach, where each discipline functions independently from the interdisciplinary approach where each discipline shares a commonly developed plan, but interacts separately with the child and parents.

26. I. S. Gilgoff and S. L. Dietrich, "Neuromuscular Diseases," in *Caring for Children with Chronic Illness: Issues and Strategies*, ed. Ruth E. K. Stein (New York: Springen Publishing Co., 1989), 184.

There are numerous models suggested for the manner of cooperation and leadership in which the collaborative physician may participate. These are each attempts to work out the functioning of a new experience of managing chronic illness in children that involves true participation in the decision-making process and not an abdication to some form of autonomy.

THE PHYSICIANS AND THEIR IMPLICIT ETHICS

Recalling once again that our work is *inductive and a work of synthesis* we proceed from the dimensions we have used to construct the ideal types of the physician to an exploration of how these three ideal types deal with ethical issues in practice. We note indicators that form the implicit ethics that guide the decision making of each type.

The Expert

Autonomy

The approach to autonomy and the advocacy of the individual practised by this physician is beneficence in the form of paternalism. Paternalism is exhibited when the physician feels justified in interfering with a person's liberty for their own good.[27] The child's good is often determined by the physician without consultation. Reasons for lack of consultation vary from time constraints to concerns about the ability of families to understand procedures or consequences, or a feeling of protection for the family. The consequence is imposed decisions.

In a discussion of care of infants with prolonged ventilator dependency, the attitude seems to be not only that the physician is the most capable of deciding what is best for the infant, the location of care is best determined by the physician for the sake of the child. The physician and the environment he controls provide "a better environment for the patient ... allowing the caretaker to focus on nutrition and cognitive, physical and social development, as well as encouraging parental bonding and support."[28] This choice for the infant is above requests from parents and others to move the child to another location such as the home.

---

27. Alan Fleischman, "Ethical Views and Values," 92.

28. E. Bancalari, "Care of the Infant with Prolonged Ventilator Dependency," *Journal of the American Medical Association* 258, no. 23 (December 18, 1987): 3430-3431.

Location of Care

Continuing with the Bancalari source noted in the preceding section on autonomy, the attitude of the Expert to location of care is expanded along the same lines. "Home care may not only contribute to the death of the child, but may create a sense of responsibility and guilt in the family."[29] Barring ideal conditions in the home, the hospital is the best place for the child. An insight into the background for this type of choice is provided in Berman's *Pediatric Decision Making* when physicians make decisions about hospital admissions. The author notes that few questions are raised about biosocial issues except in cases of chronic illnesses such as asthma, where physicians were to "assess parental attitude and the ability of the family to care for the children at home."[30] The general approach seems to be that if there is a question of parental ability, the locus of choice for care is the hospital.

Further information on the attitude of the Expert on the issues of location of care is provided from the work of Diehl on the perceptions and feelings of parents of children with complex needs. Great frustration is mentioned when it came to getting information from physicians on home care and realistic future expectations for their children. Parents also felt that there were unnecessary admissions to the hospital by physicians who would overact to the complex nature of the child's needs.

Economics

Ackerman notes that the limits of social resources, including economic ones, for pediatric care are being stretched more from technological advances that allow more children who once would have died to live and become recipients of further interventions than from strains upon the affluence of society.[31] The Expert seems generally to favour intervention with innovative technology, at least in part because of their stance in favour of technology and its application. Caplan calls for a questioning of providing aggressive care to all infants regardless of condition or prognosis, considering the strains these children may place on society in the future. This appears to suggest that while medical intervention may be desirable, there is not always a reflection beyond the intervention and its immediate effects, both for the life of the child and

---

29. Bancalari, "Care of the Infant with Prolonged Ventilator Dependency," 3431.

30. Stephan Berman, *Pediatric Decision Making* (Philadelphia: B. C. Decker, 1985), 48. See also pages 58, 86, 168 and 181 for other examples.

31. Terrence F. Ackerman, "Innovative Lifesaving Treatments: Do Children Have a Moral Right to Receive Them?" in *Contemporary Issues in Paediatric Ethics*, ed. Michael M. Burgess and Brian E. Woodrow (Lewiston: Edwin Mellen Press, 1991), 55.

the society in which the child will live. Among the factors to be considered are the economic ones.

Plante does include one method of economic decision making in discussing cost-effectiveness as a tool for making a decision about surgery for a 10-year-old. He refers to the practice of discounting of future life years when life expectancy is a measure of outcome:

> Many would argue that a year of life beginning in 20 years should still be as valuable to the individual as a year of life beginning tomorrow. In keeping with usual economic principles, however, when costs are measured in terms of dollars, future costs are discounted to model the losses or gains that alternative resource use could provide.[32]

Decision Making

From the preceding three sections on the Expert and autonomy, location of care and economics, it is evident that much of the discussion centres around decision making. This section will deal with this question specifically.

The Expert approaches decision making with two particular perspectives: power and paternalism. Physicians are obsessed with the challenge of the moment without due consideration for the long-term outcome of their interventions. "Our need to teach physicians how to save lives also contributes to our need to believe that we are morally correct in our pursuit."[33] One potential consequence is "[b]ad decisions that are sometimes well motivated come from the professional challenge of reaffirming our own omnipotence."[34] An example is provided in the approach outlined as follows:

> in recent years there has been a growing acceptance in some American hospitals of a "treat, wait, and see" approach to the dilemma of whether and when to initiate care. That is, rather than deciding immediately whether to provide or withhold all treatments, many clinicians begin treatment of imperiled newborns at birth and then make assessments later concerning continuing care.[35]

---

32. Dennis A. Plante, Seymour Zimbler and Stephen G. Pauker, "A Ten-Year-Old Boy with Cerebral Palsy and Femoral Anteversion: How Much Does It Hurt to Break a Leg?" *Medical Decision Making* 4, no. 2 (1984): 246.

33. Battle, "Beyond the Nursery Door," 419.

34. Ibid., 418.

35. Arthur L. Caplan, "Imperiled Newborns—Introduction," *Hastings Center Report* 7, no. 16 (December 1987): 5.

Such decisions are those of the treating physician's "reasonable medical judgement."[36] The Diehl article already cited noted the frustration of parents with the lack of inclusion and consultation in the decision-making process when dealing with the physician who acted alone. Echenberg notes that in significant instances the nurses involved with a patient were not consulted in decisions to place or withdraw life support.[37]

Some aspects of paternalism have already been mentioned. Fleischman situates the issue concisely:

> Medicine, particularly pediatrics, is often paternalistic: we constantly recommend treatments and courses of action to our patients, but frequently do not share the decision-making responsibility with the patient or the patient's family. Sometimes physicians arrogantly impose treatment decision rather than discussing them.[38]

Diehl notes that when a child is hospitalized frequently or for a long period, parents feel that professionals make parenting decisions without consultation.

Team Leader

Autonomy

For this physician, the best interest of the child-patient is the guiding ethical principle. The definition of best interest, however, does not seem to be the exclusive domain of the physician, although the physician appears to have the final say. The approach recognizes there may be multiple approaches to the problem and that social values need to be considered in the care of chronically ill children. Drash gives an example of this approach to autonomy for a child with juvenile diabetes.[39] The goal of physician and patient is to attain the best level of metabolic control and negotiate to achieve what is practicable. In the negotiation, however, the rules of the physician take on the proportions of commandments allowing for a reward/punishment system to fall into place. Even implicitly the physician retains the power of the rule maker.

On a theoretical level, Eaton ascribes to the pediatrician the following roles for assuring not only primary care but special services for chil-

---

36. Cynthia B. Cohen, Betty Levin and Kathy Powderly, "A History of Neonatal Intensive Care and Decisionmaking," *Hastings Center Report* 17, no. 6 (December 1987): 8.

37. Robert J. Echenberg, "Permanently Locked-In Syndrome in the Neurologically Impaired Neonate," *The Journal of Clinical Ethics* 3, no. 3 (September 1992): 208.

38. Fleischman, "Ethical Views and Values," 92.

39. Drash, "Juvenile Diabetes."

dren with chronic illness: (1) coordination of care (community resources, specialists and interdisciplinarity); (2) assessment of the child and case management; (3) assessment of the family and counselling; (4) leadership in identifying and providing child and family needs; (5) advocacy to allow child and family to participate in health care management and, on a broader scale, community education for prevention.[40] This approach allows for the involvement of numerous persons and interests in the care of a child but sees the focus not on the child and family, but rather in the coordinating role of the physician.

Location of Care

This physician is open to the possibility of care in multiple locations, including the family home. When home care is chosen, the pediatrician can take on the role of educator of parents in their quasi medical role and in resource availability. Resources include therapists and other specialists to promote "optimal development, mobility, and independence of the child."[41] The educator role is also mentioned by Lantos along with negotiation with parents in making the decision whether to send a child home.[42]

Economics

From the literature surveyed, the interest of this physician in terms of economics is in providing the family with the referrals and the resources to manage the financial strains of caring for a child at home. This includes physicians' prescriptions that allow for reimbursements to linkages with community groups that have resources.[43]

Decision Making

Consistent with attitudes outlined above, this physician approaches decision making in a collaborative manner with the best interests of the child as the motivating intention. The role of the physician on the team is very often the central one of team leader, "quarterback" or coordinator. This is an emerging challenge for the pediatrician who must interact with

---

40. A. P. Eaton, D. L. Coury and A. K. Richard, "The Roles of Professionals and Institutions," in *Caring for Children with Chronic Illness*, ed. Ruth E. K. Stein, 81.

41. David L. Coutler, Thomas H. Murray and Mary C. Cerreto, "Practical Ethics in Pediatrics," *Current Problems in Pediatrics* 18, no. 3 (March 1988): 186, 188.

42. John D. Lantos and Arthur F. Kohrman, "Ethical Aspects of Pediatric Home Care," *Pediatrics* 89, no. 5 (May 1992): 922-923.

43. See Coulter, Murray and Cerreto, "Practical Ethics in Pediatrics," 186-188. See also Cohen, Levin and Powderly, "A History of Neonatal Intensive Care and Decisionmaking," 26-28.

other specialists who are often not physicians to manage this child's developmental disabilities or problems. This central role is seen to affect the ultimate quality of the child's life.

In the literature, the teams are described as multidisciplinary or interdisciplinary often within the same paragraph and seemingly without distinction. There is evidently a degree of lack of clarity on the nature of the collaboration in which the physician is involved. There is some stress in the literature on the need for physicians to know their own values and motivations and the degree to which these and their position of power affect their decision making and interaction with other members of the health care team and the child and family.

The Collaborator

Autonomy

There is recognition by this physician that his or her contact with the child who is chronically ill and the family will consist of encounters at times of crisis. To facilitate autonomy for the child and family, the role of the physician is to educate those involved as to how to manage the situation and be available in times of crisis.[44] This physician can distinguish between the autonomy of the child and the autonomy of the family and opt for the child in instances of conflict.[45] There is also a recognition of the ability of the child to be involved in the treatment process in recognizing his or her own best interest according to developing capacity. The notion of the child giving assent to procedures is operative here.[46]

In discussing this issue concerning neuromuscular diseases, Gilgoff and Dietrich[47] write that the object of health care is to maintain the most functional state possible and to facilitate the attainment of as many life goals as possible. This is accomplished through the prevention or delay of complications in a lifestyle that is as close to normal as possible. Treatment by a physician alone cannot be justified. The ideal approach is a contractual relation between patient–parent–team that clarifies areas of responsibility. Children with chronic illness cannot be helped only by expanding the roles of physicians and other health care professionals. Children and their families need to be partners with medical personnel.

---

44. Leighton E. Cluff, "Chronic Disability of Infants and Children: A Foundation's Experience," *Journal of Chronic Disease* 38, no. 1 (1985): 122.

45. Fleischman, "Ethical Views and Values," 93.

46. Coulter, Murray and Cerreto, "Practical Ethics in Pediatrics," 155-156.

47. I. S. Gilgoff and S. L. Dietrich, "Neuromuscular Diseases," 183-195.

Location of Care

A central issue in the best location of care for a child is the degree of responsibility felt by the physician. Physicians know the risks of home care, while the parent knows the family's needs. Therefore, there is a need for education and negotiation with parents, with a recognition that reduction of risk is "consistent with the promotion of the greatest possible medical and developmental benefit for the child."[48] The physician acknowledges a spectrum of responsibility that requires assessment in each situation.

Another issue mentioned in the literature and responded to by this model of physician is sensitivity to organizing care around family needs and concerns (including racial and ethnic variables). It includes basing care in the community where the child can experience integration into the family and the neighbourhood in as great a degree as is possible. The goal of such an approach is to help prevent mental health problems, to which children with chronic illness are prone.[49]

Economics

In discussing the issue of cost-effectiveness of interventions with particular technologies, this physician does not use this mode of evaluation as a means to justify rationing nor to abdicate his or her dedication to care for a particular patient.[50] The situation of a child is neither a means for research nor a source of new information.

The discussion of economics for the physicians as Team Leaders or Collaborators is brief and the indicators of how they address this issue are sparse. The role of physician as gatekeeper is not one that is evident here.

Decision Making

Bartholome outlines the role of the physician who collaborates as providing competent care, providing accurate information to parent and child according to their ability to understand, defining treatment options clearly, stating the consequences of each treatment option, assisting parent/ child in making a responsible decision and avoiding abandoning the parent/

---

48. Lantos and Kohrman, "Ethical Aspects of Pediatric Home Care," 923.

49. J. M. Patterson and G. Geber, "Preventing Mental Health Problems in Children with Chronic Illness or Disability," Ph.D. diss., University of Minnesota, March 1992, 8.

50. Joan Venes, "Pediatric Neurosurgery: Guidelines and Cost Containment," *Pediatric Neurosurgery* 19 (1993): 5.

child after the decision is made.[51] This understanding of role and decision making emphasizes the moral, and not the technical, aspect of the professions. Bartholome also reminds physicians to be honest about the fact that nurses provide care to hospitalized infants and need to be consulted and involved in decisions about their care. These attitudes form the core of the collaborative decision making of this model:

> medicine, nursing and all the health care professions are in their practice moral, not technical, enterprises... Every decision made by a practicing health care professional that has influence on the health, welfare or life of a patient is a moral or ethical decision. Clearly all such decisions should involve and be informed by the knowledge and technology of medical science, but so-called medical science only tells us what can be done, not what ought to be done. [52]

The nature of the decision-making process also differs in this model.

Authors in the literature surveyed suggest that the best method for making decisions involving children is the one chosen by this model of physician: open, honest discussions with health care professionals and families. Decisions are best made in a collaborative, rather than prescriptive, manner, using all resources and disciplines. Another attitude is offered by Gillet: physicians are enjoined to be

> humble participants in ethical decisions, rather than pontificating judges. Our expertise as doctors stops where the medical aspects of the decision and the canons of good medical practice stop. The doctor should provide a voice of experience and even wisdom, but where medicine meets human values, he must recognize personal limits.[53]

51. William G. Bartholome, "Withholding/Withdrawing Life-Sustaining Treatment," in *Contemporary Issues in Paediatric Ethics*, ed. Michael M. Burgess and Brian E. Woodrow (Lewiston: Edwin Mellen Press, 1991), 23, 27-29, 30.

52. Bartholome, "Withholding/Withdrawing Life-Sustaining Treatment," 32.

53. Gillet, "The Ethical Challenge of Sick Children," *Pediatrician* 17 (1990): 62.

SYNTHESIS: THE PHYSICIAN AS MORAL AGENT

The Expert as Moral Authority

The Expert operates within the field of pediatric chronic care head and shoulders above others through the traditional power held by this profession. Decisions are made on his or her knowledge and experience and are carried out by others, particularly nurses. These physicians are somewhat isolated from the rest of the health care community. The implicit ethics here refers to the traditional power of the profession, a power not restricted to medical expertise, but also to the transfer of this expertise into the moral dimension. The physician is not only an expert but also one who knows what is good for others, the laypeople. This implicit ethics leads to an ethics of authority where the best interests of the child are subordinated to the standards of the authority. This physician is the guardian of the institution and expresses a conventional morality.

The Team Leader as Moral Interpreter

The Team Leader retains the traditional position of authority but recognizes and accepts as valuable the input of other players in the health care enterprise. Decisions are made after consultation and consideration of others involved, primarily those in health care, but also the family and the child. This type's implicit ethics acknowledges the limits of the authority of the Expert in favour of a search for the best interests of the child defined by multiple perspectives. The authority here is not based on technical expertise or position but rather on the service of the leader. There is a shift from reliance on codes of conduct to principles. Recognizing these principles might challenge institutions and codes.

The Collaborator as Moral Creator

The Collaborator arrives at a decision with the group after engaging in a process of consensus building. This process is complex and time-consuming while acknowledging the importance of all involved in the decision. There is here another example of a moral agent who is moral creator and recognizes the limits of medical science, as well as respects others and especially includes the child and the family.

CONCLUSION

The distinct approaches of the physicians as modelled above to the practice of care in the field of pediatric chronic illness give us insight into the manner in which each type lives certain values and the particular approach that each brings to this field. Even a cursory reading of the above information will provide one with an awareness of the potential for conflict between differing types of physicians as well as the possibility for interprofessional disagreement over roles, functions and particularly decision making. This is especially true when we consider the implicit ethics of each and their stance as moral agents, which varies from maintaining the status quo to innovation.

Physicians bring to this field a wealth of scientific and technical expertise and a tradition of power and authority. Their position is viewed as unique by the health care user. They are limited, however, in their practice and expertise by the vast quantity of information and the requirements of specialization. They are confronted with the need to share power and authority in the practice of medicine, willingly or not, with other physicians and health care providers with differing expertise.

SUMMARY CHART OF IDEAL TYPES AND IMPLICIT ETHICS OF THE PHYSICIAN IN THE FIELD OF PEDIATRIC CHRONIC ILLNESS

IDEAL TYPES AND IMPLICIT ETHICS: physicians as moral agents	ETHICAL ISSUES			
	AUTONOMY	LOCATION OF CARE	ECONOMICS	DECISION MAKING
THE EXPERT AS MORAL AUTHORITY— conventional approach to morality; authoritarian	Paternalistic— interests of the child determined by authority	Institutional and scientific interests are determining factors	Cost-benefit effectiveness	Sole decision maker; the authority
THE TEAM LEADER AS MORAL INTERPRETER— interprets values and principles	Best interests of the child negotiated with others	Multicentred where best interests of the child can be served	Openness to alternatives	Directs decisions according to the best interests of the child
THE COLLABORATOR AS MORAL CREATOR— emphasizes shared responsibility	Contractual— the child is partner	Multicentred to serve best interests of the child and shared responsibility	Cost-benefit effectiveness is broadly considered	Partner in a medical enterprise; not a pontificating judge

Chapter 4

The Social Worker as Moral Agent

Jean-Marc Larouche
and Tim Flaherty

INTRODUCTION

In the course of the literature search on nurses and physicians, the indicators drawn from professional journals and texts were collected into dimensions that gave us three ideal types of each profession with distinct approaches to ethical issues due to their distinct implicit ethics. In the course of the documentary analysis on the social worker, having used a corpus of literature comparable to that for physicians and nurses, it became evident that our discussion of the social worker would be different. First of all, it is clear that for the social worker in the field of pediatric chronic illness, there is more consensus on the nexus of the profession. Second, we noted no significant differences in the writing analyzed that would allow us to sketch more than one ideal type of social worker. We did identify four major characteristics of the social worker, and will distinguish these in the discussion of the history of the profession and in the discussion of autonomy. This will allow the reader to note the lack of distinctiveness of indicators and support the conclusion of the existence of one major ideal type. This chapter begins with a brief account of the emergence of the social worker in the field of health care. We note the major characteristics of the social worker and indicators of the one ideal type that we construct.

HISTORICAL PERSPECTIVE

The social work profession has traditionally been engaged in a commitment where concern for both the person and the person's environment is paramount.[1] Social work in a health care setting is said to have begun

---

1. Carel B. Germain, "Social Work Identity, Competence, and Autonomy: The Ecological Perspective," *Social Work in Health Care* 6, no.1 (September 1980): 1-10.

around 1905 to 1920, a period that saw the practice of social work first being established in psychiatric hospitals.[2] From the start of social work in a Boston hospital at the turn of the century, the goals of medical social work were to help patients and families deal with illness and to help them in retaining their sense of control over their lives.[3]

The period from 1905 to 1920 saw social work firmly established in health care settings.[4] Social work grew during the 1920s in response to the growth of public health progress and the need for preventive programs in the education system. By the 1930s, the influence of federal programs demanded that social work departments develop to better serve economically disadvantaged groups. Throughout the 1940s and 1950s, social workers received training in and practised a psychoanalytic approach to their work. Initiated in part by the struggle for civil liberties, social work of the 1960s emphasized social action and the need to eliminate those things that caused social and psychological dysfunction. During the 1970s and 1980s, the social work profession turned from this outward evaluation to an inward and self-oriented evaluation. During this period, the profession gathered data, developed its theoretical approaches and technical skills, and progressed toward specialization. Through increased self-awareness, public sanction and funding, the profession was able to realize a status of independence. It sought its own autonomy, rather than being dependent on physicians for guidance.[5]

Originally, social work practice in health care was intended to be a support for the physician.[6] In the late part of the nineteenth century in the United States, physicians were appointed to assist other physicians by visiting patients at home, interpreting instructions to the patient and reporting on home conditions. It was later evident that a nurse with an ability for social service was required, since not only were nurses familiar with medical practice, but at the time, it was being perceived that a patient's difficulties in his or her personal life may be the cause, and not the result, of the illness. Social work, then, attempted to focus on alleviating broader social issues. The role of the social worker became one of the

2. Abraham Lurie, "Social Work in Health Care in the Next Ten Years," *Social Work in Health Care* 2, no. 4 (June 1977): 419-428.

3. Susan J. Bendor, "The Clinical Challenge of Hospital-Based Social Work Practice," *Social Work in Health Care* 13, no. 2 (Winter 1987): 25-34.

4. Lurie, "Social Work in Health Care in the Next Ten Years," 419-428.

5. Edgar A. Perretz, "Social Work Education for the Field of Health: A Report of Findings from a Survey of Curricula," *Social Work in Health Care* 1, no. 3 (March 1976): 357-365.

6. Frances Nason, "Beyond Relationship: The Current Challenge in Clinical Practice," *Social Work in Health Care* 14, no. 4 (1990): 9-24.

"friendly visitor," who was both sympathetic toward the patient, but also paternalistic and moralistic.[7]

At first, little training was needed to work with people in this "visiting" capacity.[8] However, at the beginning of the twentieth century, the need for those who worked in human services to achieve a standard of professional education began to develop. Social work embarked on a search for legitimation, which was similar to what was occurring in medicine and nursing. From this, schools of social work emerged, offering courses in the knowledge, skills and values of social work. The set of skills and functions that specifically identified social workers was that which called for a sympathetic approach to the patient's condition. This involved assessment of the individual's environment and intervening on the patient's behalf should it become necessary. The concept of the person and his or her environment becomes very evident as a characteristic of social work concern. This perspective is especially important in promoting the maintenance and functioning of the family in cases of pediatric illness.

Medical social work was for a certain time based within a medical model of health care delivery, before directing itself as a specific field. However, once that independent status formalized, the approach of medical social work became to manage a diverse system of services that respond to the multiple aspects of problems that the patient and family face. Since the medical social worker in cases of pediatric chronic illness stands at times in relation to the patient, the family, the physicians and the hospital, the approach of the work is multidisciplinary. Social work can be regarded, for example, as a profession of collaboration, negotiation, bargaining and exchange,[9] liaison, mediation,[10] facilitation (of communication) and management (of interdisciplinary relationships).[11] This means that the social worker must posses a wide range of clinical, analytic and organizational skills.

---

7. Martin Nacman, "Social Work in Health Settings: A Historical Review," *Social Work in Health Care* 2, no. 4 (June 1977): 407-418.

8. Claire Rudolph et al., "Training Social Workers to Aid Chronically Ill Children and Their Families," in *Issues in the Care of Children with Chronic Illness: A Sourcebook on Problems, Services, and Policies*, ed. Nicholas Hobbs and James M. Perrin (San Francisco, Ca.: Jossey-Bass, 1985), 577-590.

9. Julie Abramson and Terry Mizrahi, "Strategies for Enhancing Collaboration Between Social Workers and Physicians," *Social Work in Health Care* 12, no. 1 (September 1986): 1-21.

10. Lurie, "Social Work in Health Care in the Next Ten Years," 419-428.

11. Sally E. Palmer, "Social Work in Home Dialysis: Responding to Trends in Health Care," *Social Work in Health Care* 3, no. 4 (June 1978): 363-384.

THE PROFESSIONAL IDEAL TYPE OF THE SOCIAL WORKER

Four dominant characteristics of the medical social worker arising from a review of the literature provide a context within which these skills are actualized. These are the social worker as advocate, counsellor, crisis intervener and collaborator.

As an *advocate*, the medical social worker is concerned with the rehabilitation of the patient and his or her adjustment to the environment.[12] The personal problems of the patient, the chronic illness, for example, prevent full participation in societal life and limit the realization of personal ambitions. In such a situation, the individual becomes responsible for finding solutions to the problems by receiving treatment. The social worker intervenes with expertise and therapy. The role of the social worker, then, is to defend the fundamental rights of the patient. This involves promoting treatment that improves the quality of the patient's life,[13] respects autonomy and enables the patient to achieve functioning.

As a *counsellor*, the medical social worker assesses the psychosocial aspects of the patient and his or her family.[14] This is done by exploring the feelings that the patient and the family have at the time of diagnosis and at different stages during the illness. Of primary importance is assistance in dealing with feelings of helplessness, dependency and isolation. Another clinical social work practice is to enable patients and families to maintain or strengthen their coping behaviour when faced with life- and health-threatening situations.[15]

The medical social worker as a *crisis intervener* helps patients and families cope with the trauma of the illness to master the illness instead of being controlled by it.[16] The social worker assists with family relationships and the disturbances that arise because of separation and disability.[17] In this way, social workers in the medical setting help to maintain

12. John Coates, "Ideology and Education for Social Work Practice," *Journal of Progressive Human Services* 3, no. 2 (1992): 15-30.

13. Zeev Ben-Sira, "Social Work in Health Care: Needs, Challenges and Implications for Structuring Practice," *Social Work in Health Care* 13, no. 1 (Fall 1987): 79-100.

14. Anne S. Bergman, Norman J. Lewiston and Aleda M. West, "Social Work Practice and Chronic Pediatric Illness," *Social Work in Health Care* 4, no. 3 (March 1979): 265-274.

15. Dorothy B. Black et al., "Model for Clinical Social Work Practice in a Health Care Facility," *Social Work in Health Care* 3, no. 2 (December 1977): 143-148.

16. Bendor, "The Clinical Challenge of Hospital-Based Social Work Practice," 25-34.

17. Donna Barmettler and Grace Fields, "Using the Group Method to Study and Treat Parents of Asthmatic Children," *Social Work in Health Care* 1, no. 2 (December 1975): 167-176.

individual functioning, and the functioning of the family, as they experience changes in their surroundings.

A final characteristic of the medical social worker is his or her capacity as *collaborator*. The medical social worker cooperates jointly, not only with the patient and the family, but with other health care professionals, the medical institution and representatives of other professions as well. Skill in decision making, conflict resolution and team work takes on significant importance. The social worker is also called upon frequently to provide instruction and design curricula.[18]

The literature surveyed showed that the general traits attributed to social workers are those that are applicable to social workers who practise in the field of pediatric chronic care. Attention is focussed on the child-patient and family, and on their interaction with each other and with the illness. Responses to the illness and the environment are noted and difficulties are addressed in whatever milieu they present themselves. The four characteristics sketched out above—advocate, counsellor, crisis intervener and collaborator—are almost indistinguishable from one another. We note again there is not nearly as great a distinction in the approach to the ethical issues by the social worker as was evident for the physician or for the nurse (where the distinctions are less than for the physicians). One might speculate that the recent development of social work as a distinct profession and its primarily Western formation have resulted in a greater degree of homogeneity of thought, whereas medicine and nursing have a much longer history and practice with input from diverse ages and cultures. Where distinctions exist for the social worker, they will be noted. We will therefore consider there to be one ideal type of social worker for the purposes of this chapter and will illustrate how this type deals with the four issues.

The four characteristics of the social worker as noted above function closely together, which leads us to label the ideal type of social worker as "Integrator."

SOCIAL WORKERS AND THEIR IMPLICIT ETHICS

As noted above, we find there to be one ideal type of social worker in the field of pediatric chronic illness. This one type has three predominant characteristics, which we will distinguish for the discussion of autonomy for the purpose of confirming close relationship of each in orientation and practice. This is to substantiate our conclusion that there is in fact the

---

18. L. H. Zayas and L. Dyche, "Social Workers Training Primary Care Physicians: Essential Psychosocial Principles," *Social Work* 37, no. 3 (May 1992): 1.

one type of social worker, the Integrator, which encapsulates these characteristics.

Autonomy

The Advocate

The commitment of the social worker to the child-patient's autonomy and to that of the family is evident throughout the literature. The social worker encourages children to exercise initiative and have their requests honoured to give them a sense of control and to help them battle a sense of helplessness.[19] A related issue in the same article points out how social workers sought to encourage the trust of the child by insisting they be told the truth about their situation as far as was reasonable.

The goal of the social worker as advocate is to achieve a degree of comfort with the illness by the child and the child's family that will allow them to make choices for themselves with as much freedom and self-determination as possible. This involves counselling, support and education. There is also information provided to the child and family of resources available to them to encourage their independence.[20] The social work practice of advocacy is supported by the profession's inherent holistic view.[21]

The Counsellor

The metaphor of counsellor is the principal one identified in the literature. Autonomy is consistently reinforced through the counselling process for both the child and the family. In some situations, such as a child with asthma with a psychosocial etiology, while the child encounters one phase of treatment, the social worker engages the parents in another.[22] This process is extended by the social worker to group therapy in collaboration with a psychiatrist.

---

19. Leah Beck, John K. Lattimer and Braun Esther, "Group Psychotherapy on a Children's Urology Ward," *Social Work in Health Care* 4, no. 3 (March 1979): 277.

20. Margaret Fietz, "Children with AIDS in Need of Care and Protection," *The Social Worker* 57, no. 1 (March 1989): 28.

21. Arlene M. Bregman, "Living with Progressive Childhood Illness: Parental Management of Neuromuscular Disease," *Social Work in Health Care* 5, no. 4 (June 1980): 408.

22. Barmettler and Fields, "Using the Group Method to Study and Treat Parents of Asthmatic Children," 167.

Counselling as a form of family support sorts out supportive behaviour from the destructive to build family strengths.[23] This helps to provide the child-patient with a support system within which the social worker can help overcome anxiety to develop healthy coping mechanisms, improve self-esteem and relationships, and plan realistically for the future.[24]

Counselling by the social worker also extends to the professional staff in a hospital or other institution. In times of ongoing stress when workers may lose perspective or exhibit unhealthy responses to their environment, the social worker can point out the behaviour, and may evaluate it as "normal" in the situation while being destructive of the worker's goals. The social worker may then facilitate a support group for staff.[25] A similar approach may be undertaken by social workers for recovered patients, especially long-term cancer survivors, who have particular issues to deal with in their adult lives.[26]

The Crisis Intervener

An example of this portrait of the social worker intervening to develop autonomy is given in an article by Bowden and Hopwood.[27] Dramatic intervention is required in identifying and treating psychosocial dwarfism requiring the separation of parent and child for treatment. The article suggests that it be up to social work to identify more "benign" methods of treatment and intervention geared toward change and a period for catch-up by the child.

A second example comes from Guendelman.[28] An immigrant family with a hospitalized child is further fragmented by a lack of understanding of local customs and possibilities. When no extended family is available, the child-patient or the children in the home, as well as employment and financial obligations, may become neglected. In a situation of extreme

---

23. Bregman, "Living with Progressive Childhood Illness," 407.

24. Barbara S. Finley, Carol S. Crouthamel and Robert A. Richman, "A Psychosocial Intervention Program for Children with Short Stature and Their Families" *Social Work in Health Care* 7, no. 1 (September 1981): 29.

25. Carol K. Mahan, Joan C. Krueger and Richard L. Schreiner, "The Family and Neonatal Intensive Care," *Social Work in Health Care* 7, no. 4 (June 1982): 73-74.

26. Judith W. Ross, "The Role of the Social Worker with Long Term Survivors of Childhood Cancer and Their Families," *Social Work in Health Care* 7, no. 4 (June 1982): 11-12.

27. Leora Bowden and Nancy J. Hopwood, "Psychosocial Dwarfism: Identification, Intervention and Planning," *Social Work in Health Care* 7, no. 3 (March 1982): 34.

28. Sylvia Guendelman, "Developing Responsiveness to the Health Needs of Hispanic Children and Families," *Social Work in Health Care* 8, no. 4 (June 1983): 5, 6.

distress, the social worker intervenes to provide support and information on available services.

The Collaborator

As we have seen, the social worker may collaborate with a psychiatrist to promote autonomy and coping skills with children and parents. A broader approach to collaboration is outlined by Finley, Crouthamel and Richman. Here the social worker works with a multidisciplinary team of varied individuals and fulfils the roles of program coordinator and counsellor. This position is in recognition of "skills in individual, family, group and community intervention, as well as methods and diagnosis."[29] Social workers are responsible for developing programs of collaboration where none exist and ensuring they are multidisciplinary.

Location of Care

The primary involvement of the social worker in this ethical issue is in terms of discharge planning or the determination of the most appropriate location for care of the child. It does not appear possible to distinguish the approach of social workers under one metaphor from another. In the discharge scenario it is a large process of collaboration involving child, family, caregivers, community resources and government agencies. The social worker must purposefully develop this network to receive varied ideas and suggestions and to make final decisions with the child and family. A special contribution of the social worker to this process is to openly deal with disagreement that appears during the information gathering and decision making.

Economics

As with location of care, the ethical issues surrounding economics are approached by all the portraits of social workers in a similar manner. This is perhaps because issues around economics are closely linked to location of care. It is accepted that care for the chronically ill is less expensive, and for many children more beneficial, if carried out in a home environment. Social workers recognize the economic costs of health care for families and society and accept a responsibility for equitable allocation of resources. In order not to "waste" good hospital care, social workers need to make use of community resources to avoid rehospitalization resulting from less than adequate home care.[30]

---

29. Finley Crouthamel and Richman, "A Psychosocial Intervention Program," 30.

30. Wilma Gurney, "Building a Collaborative Network," *Social Work in Health Care* 1, no. 2 (Winter 1975): 186.

Decision Making

As might be expected with near consensus in each social worker portrait on the ethical issues discussed, the issue of decision making is also approached uniformly. The social worker engages decision making as a process requiring interdisciplinary, patient-centred consultation to achieve their ultimate goal: "to work with the health care system to enable the patient to achieve the highest possible level of functioning."[31] The process of decision making involves advocacy for the family and child, counselling and intervention with all participants, and education with a feel for conflict resolution and tools for appropriate dialogue.

SYNTHESIS: THE SOCIAL WORKER AS MORAL AGENT

The Social Worker (the Integrator) as Moral Creator

The differences between the approaches of social workers outlined in this section are minimal. There is, in effect, one "ideal type" for this profession, which we label "the Integrator." Again we note this unity is most likely because of the relatively short history and evolution of social work. There is a homogeneous implicit ethics for the social worker, who is person-oriented. This orientation calls attention to the real impact of explicit ethics, codes, and institutional regulations and standards upon persons and families and the broader community. The social worker promotes an ethics of shared responsibility untied from traditional constraints and as such is a moral creator.

Decisions are seen as best made with input from all players, including those outside of the chronic care institution or hospital. This is a distinct difference from physicians and nurses, who tend to operate within the institutional boundaries. The broadly inclusive scope of the social worker brings more information to the table, both complicating and facilitating the decision-making process.

---

31. Bergman, Lewiston and West, "Social Work Practice and Chronic Pediatric Illness," 173.

CONCLUSION

The social worker brings to the health care enterprise a recently developed perspective that lacks much of the baggage of traditional constraints. This allows for new ideas and practices to be added to those already engaged in the care of children with chronic illness. Coming from the field of social sciences, this profession is not constrained by the narrow framework of outcomes and strategy presented by medicine. The broader perspective is one of possibilities. This asset of the social worker is also its greatest liability. Medicine, in particular, while accepting technical and scientific advances, is not noted for acceptance of social change or structural change. The social worker is thus in the position of having to demonstrate the value of their profession for more than picking up work discarded by other professions.

SUMMARY CHART OF IDEAL TYPES AND IMPLICIT ETHICS OF THE SOCIAL WORKER IN THE FIELD OF PEDIATRIC CHRONIC ILLNESS

IDEAL TYPE AND IMPLICIT ETHICS:	ETHICAL ISSUES			
social workers as moral agents	AUTONOMY	LOCATION OF CARE	ECONOMICS	DECISION MAKING
THE SOCIAL WORKER AS INTEGRATOR/ MORAL CREATOR— emphasizes shared responsibility and broad inclusion	Ordered to full functioning of the child and family	Best interests of the child, family and community	Best interests of the child, family and community	Shared responsibility

Chapter 5

Synthesis of Part 1

Jean-Marc Larouche
and Tim Flaherty

The objective of this part of the study was to use the tools of ideal type, a "portrait," to provide the background to examine both the ways in which conflicts of values are lived and the ways in which ethical decisions are made in long-term care units of pediatric hospitals. The most fruitful result of this documentary research has come as *insights* into the professional interaction of physicians, nurses and social workers. This interaction is considered on both intraprofessional and interprofessional levels.

PROFESSIONAL INTERACTION

Analysis of professional interaction shows three points of interest:

1. It is significant to note that in sketching the portraits in the three preceding chapters, the distinctions in portraits between physicians and nurses were much more evident than those for social workers. The degree of distinction was greatest for the physicians to the point of being mutually exclusive as, for example, with the physician as Expert and the physician as Collaborator. This suggests the possibility of intraprofessional conflict that may exist before involvement with other professionals. Nurses face a similar problem. As noted, they exhibit no common understanding of roles such as "Advocate," where definitions vary from a legal mode of rights protection against incompetent others in health care to a philosophical promotion of the existential self. There is a level of conflict suggested here that may arise from confusion more than disagreement. Social workers present a more united philosophical and practical front. There seems to be a more common understanding of professional goals and standards of practice. Although there is some evidence of a hierarchy within social

work itself, conflicts from this source are minimal in the literature surveyed.

2. In the area of interprofessional interaction, a significant indicator is found in the number of references made by each profession of the others in the literature database prepared for this documentary analysis. The numbers tell an interesting story. In the "physician" database, nurses are mentioned in seven of 114 texts consulted; social workers are mentioned in two texts. The "nurse" database mentions physicians in 38 of 145 texts and social workers in three. The social worker database, on the other hand, includes mention of physicians in 95 of 107 texts and nurses in 19. The suggestion raised by these numbers falls into the area of collaboration. If the number of references is low, is it an indicator of the true nature of collaboration or is it an indicator of one profession's evaluation of another? If the number is high, is it an indicator of an effort of inclusion in collaboration or an indicator of the social reality of the hierarchical structure of the health care enterprise? These are questions for further research.

3. The third area of interest in professional interaction is suggested by each profession's approach to hierarchy in health care. By tradition and in the literature surveyed, physicians see themselves, for the most part, as leading the medical hierarchy. Where professional interaction is acknowledged, it is (except in some texts that provide indicators of the physician as Collaborator) understood that the physician is leader or in charge. The literature on nursing seems to acknowledge this view. Nurses appear to challenge this indirectly in practice through adopting the role as Coordinator, which moves all players on to a more level playing field. Evidently, nurses have adopted this role because they see themselves as the most qualified for the role due to their particular skills and their consistent presence in all levels of medical care for children. These qualifications are acknowledged among the other portraits only by the physician as Collaborator.

Social work presents a very different understanding of the medical hierarchy. Social workers very clearly see themselves as the most qualified to coordinate collaboration and case management. The rationale for this position is their unique position in health care. Although non-medical in orientation, they have adopted medical language for their practice. Social workers diagnose, treat and assess patients. They offer therapy as well as counselling. Social workers see part of their role in the education of physicians and nurses in formal settings and curriculum development for these professions. They also include among their qualifications the social science background, which they perceive as having broader and more patient-centred goals than medicine or nursing. Social workers see themselves possessing unfettered allegiance to the client. It is also interesting to note that social workers are the most explicit in acknowledging the reality of interprofessional conflict and count among their skills those of conflict resolution.

IMPLICIT ETHICS

In our discussion of the nurse and the physician we have observed a shift from conventional ethics, which refers to institutions and codes of conduct, to a post-conventional ethics, which refers to values and a process of shared responsibility. The move from authority to responsibility in deliberation in the field of pediatric chronic illness represents a transformation of ethics. This transformation is accompanied by an evolution in the professions and seems to follow an evolution that we observe in the larger society engaged in the moral enterprise. From the moral reproducer, which functions as conservator of stability and predictability as the highest value, we observe the emergence of those who begin to break from this as they operate as moral interpreters of codes and standards. A third group of professionals functions as moral creators looking to *innovative strategies for interaction and decision making.*

In the field of pediatric chronic care we noted the way in which the professionals involved addressed four ethical themes or issues identified in earlier research as central issues. Of these, two issues—economics and location of care—were the focus of less attention by the professionals involved in the clinical setting. Regulation and policy in economics and location of care are usually "givens" in the clinical setting and therefore the decisions are made by others outside of the clinical team. They do not ignore these issues but recognize the limits of their professional influence. One exception to this may be the Expert, who may not conform to institutional guidelines when making decisions based on his or her determination of the best interests of his or her patient on a case by case basis.

The issues of autonomy and decision making are two very important issues that the professionals considered engage seriously. There is recognition that in these two areas in particular, clinical decisions do have a substantial impact. In particular, the professionals considered place emphasis on the issue of autonomy, an issue with which they live on a daily basis and over which they have some power and control.

Conclusion

From the analysis of the literature considered, professionals involved in decision making in the field of pediatric chronic illness are concerned with the process of decision making and the ethical issue of patient autonomy in particular. The literature also revealed that value conflicts among physicians, nurses and social workers active in the field of pediatric chronic illness appear on three levels:

1. the intraprofessional level, where there are varied understandings of each profession's role, goals and place in the health care enterprise;

2. the interprofessional level, where there are varied understandings of the role, goals and value of other professionals in the health care enterprise; and

3. the collaborative or cooperative level, where the conflicts from the two preceding levels remain unacknowledged or unresolved, and meaningful collaboration is impeded by further conflict.

The conflict of values noted on these three levels relates to conflicts rooted in the differences in the implicit ethics within each profession as well as between professions and others involved in the health care enterprise. From Moral Authority or Reproducer to Moral Creator, there is a broad difference in values and interpretation of meaning. Attempts to address conflict must consider the difference in the implicit ethics of those involved, as these seem to be more in conflict than the explicit ethics of codes and standards.

There are two major directions for research within the scope of this present study. The first is the need for assessment of findings in terms of stability over time and in the field of clinical practice, on actual long-term care units in pediatric hospitals. The second is the development of a means of addressing the conflicts that arise in health care teams, both in terms of function and goal clarification. These two directions will be considered in the following parts.

PART 2

**ETHICAL DELIBERATION:
THEORETICAL PERSPECTIVES FROM THE
FIELDS OF ETHICS AND CONFLICT STUDIES**

Introduction to Part 2

Kenneth R. Melchin

Currently, health care practitioners who must wrestle with ethical issues in their daily work experience are confronted with a diversity of theories and principles in the field of ethics. Professionals do not have a standardized set of ethical tools and methods for deliberating and deciding on issues. Rather, they must choose among diverse sets of such tools. Furthermore, their own personal choices are never the last word. They must work with other professionals whose approaches to ethics are often quite different. These differences often give rise to conflicts. In health care institutions, these conflicts often must be resolved through discourse among the various professionals involved in health care practice.

This situation is not unique to health care. To an ever-increasing degree, researchers in ethics are turning their attention to the analysis of ethical discourse and are developing theories on how the process of discourse can be guided to yield constructive dialogue amid conflicting ethical convictions. Many are finding that even when interlocutors differ on ethical issues, they can still find common agreements about the procedures and goals of the discourse that will allow them to work through issues toward mutually acceptable action strategies.

While the field of ethics has been turning its attention to the process of discourse, the field of conflict resolution has been developing theories and practical tools for the analysis and management of conflicts in diverse spheres of life. The goal of the second part of this study is to draw upon published literature in ethical theory and conflict resolution to develop a coherent theoretical perspective on ethical deliberation and to develop practical tools that can help health care professionals in the deliberation process in multiprofessional teams. To do this, we draw upon the work of the Canadian philosopher-theologian Bernard Lonergan for the ethical theory framework for synthesizing the contributions from these diverse fields of research.

Chapter 6, by James Sauer, presents a brief survey of the field of discourse ethics, identifies two main lines of theory in this field and proposes an argument for drawing on both lines of theory for a comprehensive understanding of ethical discourse. Chapter 7, by Kenneth R. Melchin, introduces the ethical theory of Bernard Lonergan to develop a framework for introducing contributions from discourse ethics and conflict resolution into ethical deliberation in health care. Chapter 8, by Peter Monette, surveys research contributions in conflict resolution and draws upon the work of Lonergan to propose a set of insights for applying conflict resolution to ethical deliberation in health care teams.

Chapter 6

Theories of Discourse Ethics

James Sauer

One of the fundamental assumptions of the liberal tradition of democracy, and so of the institutions nourished explicitly or implicitly by
that tradition, is that there are a plurality of values that can conflict with
one another and that are not reducible to one another. Consequently, it is
widely accepted that value conflicts will not be eliminated. We do not
expect to resolve our value conflicts to the satisfaction of all parties.[1]
However, this belief sets up a problem for social living. How can this
irreducible pluralism of values be combined with a notion of legitimate
social or collective action? Does collective action not require a common
commitment to value?

In the past two decades, a set of positions has emerged in philosophy
that argues that the structure of discourse can provide a framework for
grounding or validating fundamental norms and values. The various positions are based on the recognition that values justification is part of the
rational process of argumentation and that argumentation is a subspecies
of discourse. Therefore, discourse, viewed procedurally or contextually,
provides the potential for grounding moral judgments.[2]

This turn to discourse in ethics is an effort to reframe traditional philosophical questions about moral knowledge into questions about moral

---

1. Bernard Williams, "Conflicts of Value," in *Moral Luck: Philosophical Papers, 1973-1980* (Cambridge: Cambridge University Press, 1981), 71- 82, puts forward an excep-
   tionally well reasoned version of this thesis.

2. Obviously this is a subspecies of the problem of justification of moral claims. There is
   no value going into the labyrinths of this discussion. A short well-documented discussion is provided by Tom Beauchamp, *Philosophical Ethics: An Introduction to Moral
   Philosophy* (New York: McGraw-Hill, 1992), 81-92. Douglas Odegard, ed., *Ethics
   and Justification* (Edmonton: Academic Printing and Publishing, 1988), provides a
   collection of recent essays in the field.

discourse.[3] In this shift, epistemological questions about the relationship between rational, knowing subjects and a rational, knowable objective morality are not the primary focus of concern. The new aim is to understand morality as a socially embedded practice where the crucial questions are those that have to do with the way the meaning and legitimacy of moral beliefs and values are established, reinterpreted and transformed within the discourse acts of a culture.[4]

This reframing of the traditional question of ethics has opened up to new philosophical scrutiny the relationship between morality as private commitment and morality as public action.[5] If the tradition of liberal democracy has been to view ethics merely as a personal, private affair, the turn to discourse has shed light on the public dimension of morality. This, in turn, has contributed to a new examination of the private–public nexus of social interaction.[6]

DISCOURSE ETHICS: TWO DISTINCTIVE APPROACHES

The field of discourse ethics can be divided into two general approaches, each with spokespersons in Europe and North America. We will use the terms "proceduralists" and "contextualists" to describe these two approaches. The focus of the proceduralists is the structure of discourse and the norms and obligations that flow from the analysis of this structure, which are binding on rational interlocutors, regardless of the content of the value claims. The focus of the contextualists is the cultural context of meanings, which sets the reference frame for both the rules

---

3.   Seyla Benhabib, "In the Shadow of Aristotle and Hegel: Communicative Ethics and Current Controversies in Practical Philosophy," *The Philosophical Forum* 21 (1989-1990), 1-31.

4.   See Stuart Hampshire, *Morality and Conflict* (Oxford: Basil Blackwell, 1983), 2, 79, 94 *ff.*

5.   On the relationship of morality and ethics, see James E. Rachels, *The Elements of Moral Philosophy* (New York: McGraw-Hill, 1990), 3-5. Rachels argues that moralities are the praxiological "codes" or "frameworks" of moral reasoning that human beings employ to guide conduct. Ethics is a systematic reflection on the adequacy, soundness, issues and problems of these positions in a public forum governed by reason. Paul Ricoeur insists that ethics, which reconstructs the sources of moral imperatives in human intentionality and action, comes before morality, which is concerned with the formal notions of the norms of permission and interdiction. See Paul Ricoeur, "Avant la loi morale: L'éthique," in *Encyclopaedia Universalis,* vol. 22 (Paris, 1985), 42, 44-45. We will not resolve these differences here. What is important is the recognition of the self–world connection in ethics through a notion of reasons about actions.

6.   See Jean-Marc Larouche, "Des sciences morales à une éthique des sciences de la morale et de l'éthique," *Ethica* 5, no. 2 (1993): 9-30.

and the content of the discourse. Debates between representatives of the two approaches have taken quite different directions on the two continents. However, in spite of these differences, there have been signs of mutual recognition that warrant the twofold division.

In Europe, the two approaches are represented by the communicative ethics of Jürgen Habermas (proceduralists) and the hermeneutic philosophy of Hans-Georg Gadamer (contextualists).[7] In North America, the proceduralists are represented by the liberal theorists John Rawls and Bruce Ackerman, and the contextualists are represented by the communitarians Alasdair MacIntyre and Michael Sandel.[8] Habermas, Rawls and Ackerman have acknowledged the similarity of their projects as directed to identifying the procedural rules of public discourse. The hermeneutic philosophers and communitarians both draw on a neo-Aristotelian or virtue ethics tradition in which the contextual normativity of traditions of ethical reflection emerges as the key to understanding public discourse.

The purpose of this chapter is to organize this "talk about discourse" by considering the positions as they have developed in relation to one another. What we are interested in is how representative contributors to this conversation understand the relationship of "private" and "public" spheres of meaning and value; how, if at all, conflicts of values (or interests) can be resolved; and the significance of the notion of dialogical consensus that has come to the fore in applied ethics as an important

---

7. The primary literature on this debate is found in Jürgen Habermas, "A Review of Gadamer's *Truth and Method*," in *Understanding and Social Inquiry*, ed. F. Dallmayr and T. McCarthy (Notre Dame: University of Notre Dame Press, 1977), 335-363; *idem*, "On Systematically Distorted Communication," *Inquiry* 13 (1970): 205-218; Hans-Georg Gadamer, "On the Scope and Function of Hermeneutical Reflection," in *Philosophical Hermeneutics* (Berkeley: University of California Press, 1976), 18-43; *idem*, "Replik," in *Hermeneutik und Ideologikritik*, ed. Karl-Otto Apel (Frankfort-am-Main: Surkamp, 1971), 45-57. For a helpful critical appraisal of this debate, see Paul Ricoeur, "Ethics and Culture: Habermas and Gadamer in Dialogue," in *Political and Social Essays*, ed. S. Stewart and J. Bien (Athens: Ohio University Press, 1974), 243-270 (also published in *Philosophy Today* 17 [1973]: 153-165); *idem*, "Hermeneutics and the Critique of Ideology," in *Hermeneutics and the Human Sciences*, ed. and trans. J. B. Thompson (Cambridge: Cambridge University Press, 1982), 63-100.

8. Alasdair MacIntyre, *Whose Justice? Which Rationality?* (Notre Dame: University of Notre Dame Press, 1988); Charles Sandel, *Liberalism and the Limits of Justice* (Cambridge: Cambridge University Press, 1982); John Rawls, "Justice as Fairness: Political not Metaphysical," *Philosophy and Public Affairs* 14 (1985): 223-251; Bruce Ackerman, *Social Justice and the Liberal State* (New Haven: Yale University Press, 1980). A helpful symposium volume of essays on both sides of this debate is R. Bruce Douglass, Gerald M. Mara and Henry S. Richardson, eds. *Liberalism and the Good* (London: Routledge, 1990).

criteria of ethical justification in the public sphere.[9] In order to do this we must deal with two positions with four partners. One side is a procedural approach represented by liberalism and critical theory. The other is a contextual or substantive approach represented by various strains of communitarianism.

Alasdair MacIntyre sets up one side of the debate by arguing that all reasoning takes place within the context of some traditional mode of thought that transcends through criticism and invention the limitations of what had hitherto been reasoned in that tradition.[10] In this contextualist view, consensus is the shared understandings, values, meanings and commitment that exist in shared traditions that are prior to any moral conversation.

Habermas sets up the alternate position by arguing that traditions are systematically distorted and a philosophical program of discourse analysis must start with removing the elements of systematic distortion of self-understanding that are communicated linguistically in order to recover individual and social identity. Through self-reflective consciousness, one realizes "communicative competence." Through such competence, one is enabled beyond all distinctions to communicate, talk reciprocally and attain consensus. In this proceduralist view, consensus is an agreement that emerges among individuals who have access to particular moral conversations.

COMMUNICATIVE ETHICS: DISCOURSE AND IMPARTIALITY

Discourse or communicative ethics is an attempt to define the formal rules and communicative presuppositions that make it possible for participants in a practical discourse to arrive at a valid, rational consensus on social norms. According to Habermas, both theoretical and practical discourses are argumentative enterprises in which claims of truth

9. See, for example, Joseph Agassi, "The Logic of Consensus and of Extremes," in *Freedom and Rationality: Essays in Honor of John Watkins*, ed. Fred D'Agostino and I. C. Jarvie (Boston: Boston University Press, 1989), 3-21; Peter Caws, "Committees and Consensus: How Many Heads Are Better Than One?" *Journal of Medicine and Philosophy* 16, no. 4 (1991): 375-391; Amy Gutmann and David W. Thompson, "Moral Conflict and Political Consensus," *Ethics* 101 (1990): 64-88; Bruce Jennings, "Possibilities of Consensus: Toward Democratic Moral Discourse," *Journal of Medicine and Philosophy* 16, no. 4 (1991): 447-468; Rosemarie Tong, "The Epistemology and Ethics of Consensus: Uses and Misuses of 'Ethical' Experts," *Journal of Medicine and Philosophy* 16, no. 4 (1991): 409-426.

10. Alasdair MacIntyre, *After Virtue: An Essay in Moral Philosophy* (Notre Dame: University of Notre Dame Press, 1988), 222.

and rightness are tested and contested through the invocation of validating reasons.[11] A practical discourse aims at a rationally motivated
consensus on norms. The goal of discourse ethics is to articulate the
formal, objective and universal criteria that guide practical discourses
and that serve as the standard for distinguishing between legitimate and
illegitimate normative claims.[12]

This process, Habermas argues, is not an abstraction that is limited
to personal morality. It serves the social or public purpose of prescribing
impartiality and general reciprocity. "Impartial judgment reflects a principle which requires that in assessing interests every participant must assume the perspective of all others."[13] This means that a norm "can claim
validity only if all those potentially affected can consent to this validity
as participants of a practical discourse."[14] This emphasis on universal inclusion and consensual validity is directed to the problem of pluralism
and cooperative social action.

In attempting to specify the criteria that guide practical discourses,
discourse ethics consists of two core affirmations. The first specifies the
necessary conditions for coming to a legitimate rational agreement. The
second articulates the possible contents on a formal level of such an agreement. Procedures have a higher priority than substantive content, because
it is through the procedural rules that consensus, which legitimates a position, is established.[15] A norm of action can be considered legitimate
only if all those possibly affected would, as participants in a practical
discourse, arrive at an agreement that such a norm should come into or
remain in force.

What is to be considered as a rationally motivated agreement, however, has rather demanding preconditions. In order that all affected have
an effective equality of opportunity to assume dialogical "roles," there
must be a mutual and reciprocal recognition, without constraint, of all
autonomous rational subjects whose claims will be acknowledged if they
are supported by valid arguments.[16] That is, it must be (1) a fully public

---

11. Jürgen Habermas, "Discourse Ethics: Notes on a Programme of Philosophical Justifi-
    cation," in *The Communicative Ethics Controversy*, ed. S. Benhabib and F. Dallmayr
    (Cambridge: MIT Press, 1990), 64-65.

12. See Thomas McCarthy, *The Critical Theory of Jürgen Habermas* (Cambridge: MIT
    Press, 1978), 272-357.

13. Habermas, "Discourse Ethics," 70.

14. Ibid., 71.

15. Jürgen Habermas, "A Reply to My Critics," in *Habermas: Critical Debates*, ed. John
    B. Thompson and David Held (Cambridge: MIT Press, 1982), 254.

16. Karl-Otto Apel, *Towards the Transformation of Philosophy*, trans. Glyn Adey and David
    Frisby (London: Routledge and Kegan Paul, 1980), 227, 258-259.

communicative process free of political or economic power; and (2) it must be public in terms of access. Anyone capable of speech and action who potentially will be affected by the norms under dispute must be able to participate in the discussion on equal terms. In addition to these procedural rules regulating the organization of interaction, participants must also be able to shift, alter or change the agenda. In a practical discourse, nothing can be out of bounds or taboo, including the reserves of power, wealth, tradition or authority. The principles of procedural validity permit everyone a fair hearing and so it becomes possible to discern whether there is indeed a common interest that can become the basis of a consensus.

At the heart of discourse ethics is the desire to provide a formal principle of legitimacy for societies that are pluralistic and composed of individuals with distinct and different concepts of the "good" life. There is no basis for assuming either the absence of difference or the absence of change. No consensus, no matter how unanimous or long-lasting, is permanent. Every consensus is only empirical and so open to challenge and revision. Thus, moral consciousness, differing ways of life, values and experiments with new ways must all be granted autonomy from the mere consensus on what is just. That is, discourse ethics tries to assure the fairness of argumentation once the terms and relations of community (fundamental values) are fixed. This is to argue that fundamental values are not objects of discussion.

While conflicts involving fundamental values cannot be resolved, such resolution is not necessary in a model of communicative ethics. What is required is that the compromises be considered fair in the sense that the rules regulating such discourse are themselves open to debate and are, in principle, capable of general agreement at a deeper level of justification. At this deeper level, debates about basic constitutional rights or the preferred design of legal and political institutions are less suitably the subject matter of a fair compromise or majority rule, since it is in the context of these rights and institutions that the other rules of decision making are held to be fair. Methodological procedures of discourse are meant to institutionalize (stabilize, make normative) the rules governing fairness and impartiality.

LIBERALISM: DIALOGUE AND NEUTRALITY

Concern for impartiality and fairness is at the heart of liberalism's contribution to the dialogue-ethics connection. But liberal theory starts from a different initial position than Habermas, because basic liberal mistrust of institutions leads liberal theory to privilege the individual over the institutionalized structures of cooperative intersubjectivity.

The central feature of contemporary liberalism is its assertion of the priority of the right over the good. The principal ground for this claim is the belief that questions of right or justice should outweigh or trump considerations of social utility or the common good, thereby securing for individuals a domain of thought and action free from intrusion by others. Individuals have a right to develop freely their own identities and, in turn, to participate in the democratic process as autonomous citizens. Thus, many liberal rights impose limits or constraints on the pursuit of private and public interests, while other rights are intended to secure or render more effective the participation of individual citizens in shaping or defining the common good or democratic will.[17] The net effect of such rights is to remove certain items from the agenda of collective decision making or majority rule.[18]

Bruce Ackerman provides an illustrative example of the way liberal theory dichotomizes human living in the private sphere of commitment, conviction and choice, and in the public sphere of responsible social order. In personal dialogue, conviction is paramount for action. In public dialogue, conviction is an impediment to consensus.[19] Thus, Ackerman goes down a well-travelled road to argue that there is a disjunction or irreconcilable dissimilarity between personal morality as conviction and social ethics as a responsible social order. Ackerman describes the relationship in this way, "In ... [the] exercise of liberal conversation, P is not trying to convince the not-P's to change their minds and see the compelling truth of P. Instead, the conversation has a more pragmatic intention. It recognizes that neither P nor not-P is going to win the moral argument to the other's satisfaction, and proceeds to consider the way they might live together despite this ongoing disagreement."[20]

To meet the demands of coexistence, social partners are required to exercise "conversational restraint." Conversational restraint means that when two people disagree about some specific point, but wish to continue talking about the more general problem they wish to solve, each should prescind from the beliefs that the other rejects (1) in order to construct an argument on the basis of his or her beliefs that will convince the

---

17. John Rawls, "The Basic Liberties," in *Liberty, Equality, and Law*, ed. S. McMurrin (Salt Lake City: University of Utah Press, 1987), 3-87.

18. John Rawls, "The Idea of Overlapping Consensus," *The Oxford Journal of Legal Studies* 7 (1987): 237.

19. Bruce Ackerman, "Why Dialogue?" *Journal of Philosophy* 56 (1989): 5.

20. Ackerman, "Why Dialogue?" 10.

other of the truth of the disputed belief, or (2) in order to shift to another aspect of the problem where the possibility of agreement seems greater.[21]

The heart of the liberal notion of public dialogue is a notion of social consensus based on the least substantive content possible. Whatever values are consented to in this fashion must be neutral (or impartial) with regard to particular substantive conceptions of the good, so that the state or social institutions that incorporate values into law and policy do not destroy the individual's freedom to pursue his or her own good according to his or her own means. By bracketing moral argument until some sort of lowest possible denominator of value is reached, Ackerman hopes to identify a kind of metaconsensus on the basis of which institutions facilitating agreement or consensus can be supported.

Dialogue legitimates political discourse without in itself legitimating any particular political claim. Particular claims are legitimated by consensual agreement arrived at through dialogue. But it must be noted that the consensus, like consensus in discourse ethics, is procedural.

Ackerman uses his notion of conversational restraint to avoid the most difficult issues of conflict resolution by reducing the number of points of potential conflict. Conversational restraint means that while anything may be the object of discussion, everything is not profitable for discussion. This means that the dialogue occasioned by disagreement controls the agenda which is guided by the commitment to the largest possible scope of individual action.

COMMUNITARIANISM: DIALOGUE AND CONTEXT

The model of communitarian ethics neither assumes nor requires that most practical discourses will have a unanimous agreement as their outcome. For example, a public debate (discourse) about such policies as welfare or affirmative action may well have little chance of ending in general agreement. What is central is the moral act of dialogue itself in the formation of moral communities.

According to Alasdair MacIntyre, who exhibits a typical communitarian position, moral reflection is a type of ongoing conversation. This conversation, he argues, is structured by the embeddedness of meaning in history and tradition, because "we cannot characterize behaviour independently of intention, and we cannot characterize intentions independently

---

21. See Ackerman, "Why Dialogue?" 16; *Social Justice in the Liberal State*, 9; "Neutralities," in *Liberalism and the Good*, ed. R. B. Douglass, G. M. Mara and H. S. Richardson (New York: Routledge, 1990), 37. Also see parallel of "rational dialogue" in Charles Larmore, *Patterns of Moral Complexity* (Cambridge: Cambridge University Press, 1987), 53.

of the settings that make those intentions intelligible to the agents them-selves and to others."[22] Understanding requires understanding the con-text, because action itself has a basically historical character.[23]

What is true of the individual as agent is also true of the context in which one is embedded—the tradition. There is, we might say, a prior sociocultural consensus in a tradition that precedes (and in fact makes possible) any public discourse. A living tradition (as opposed to a dead tradition) is not one in which there is an absence of conflict; indeed, tra-ditions embody conflict because in any tradition there is continuous argu-ment about what the good is. Thus, a tradition is a historically extended, socially embodied argument about the goods that constitute the tradition.[24]

Formal argumentation and procedural validation are only one move-ment in a more complex set of human intentions and transactions. Valid-ity or legitimacy, for MacIntyre, is the social validity constituted by the ongoing historical vitality of traditions. Consensus, in this sense, is not a consensus on procedures, a minimal content of shared values, or social utility, but a consensus of common meanings and shared values out of which a common good is created by virtue of individuals aspiring to such a good in which the shared intention of the participants to talk to one another becomes the foundation of moral discourse.[25]

WHAT ARE THE ISSUES?

This cursory and admittedly unnuanced sketch of the positions still allows one to draw the central issues together and so join these debates as a single discourse about discourse. Several issues emerge as important and significant.

First, critical theory and communitarianism shared a common aversion to the idea that the individual is constituted prior to all social interaction,

---

22. MacIntyre, *After Virtue*, 206.

23. Ibid., 212.

24. Ibid., 222.

25. Continuing this conversation requires moving to the philosophy of action. While the next section of this chapter will open this field, a full exploration of the elements and arguments in the field will carry this essay too far afield. However, an excellent intro-duction to the field is provided by Carlos Moya, *Philosophy of Action: An Introduc-tion* (London: Polity Press, 1990). An older, but useful survey of the field is found in Lawrence Davis, *Theory of Action* (Englewood Cliffs, N.J.: Prentice-Hall, 1979). For applications of two contributors to this field of ethics, see Stuart Hampshire, *Thought and Action* (London: Penguin, 1990 [1959]); and Hector-Neri Castenada, "Imperatives, Decisions, and 'Oughts,'" in *Morality and the Language of Conduct*, ed. Hector-Neri Castenada and G. Nakhnikien (Detroit: Wayne State University Press, 1963), 219-299.

which is implicit in all contract theories of society, in natural rights theory and in the methodological individualistic epistemology of liberalism.

At the same time, however, Habermas has subscribed to many of the liberal views that the communitarians criticize. Like the liberal theorists, he tries through his procedural approach to ground norms without pre-judging questions of values. Unlike the liberals, however, he abandons natural rights theory and the contractarian perspective in favour of a communicative theory based on the notion of rational consent. His approach leads him to transpose into the realm of theory the "art of separation" that liberals practise in the sphere of public praxis.

Communitarians, conversely, want to bridge or minimize the gap between descriptive and evaluative expressions between the right and the good, between the grounding of norms and their application. They are unwilling to pay the price Habermas pays for universality. Their attacks are directed against the formalistic bias typical of liberal theories. They regard procedural formalism as a pretension. One cannot, they argue, generate norms, rules, institutions and principles that are neutral with regard to value, culture or historical context. They reject the belief that there is any core of procedures that any actor, no matter how situated, must accept as valid and universal.

The proceduralist view of society is that social interaction is "held together" by the "shared rules of the game," which can be agreed to by individuals and groups who hold diverse ideas as to what the game is about. Communitarians affirm the context-specific nature of the validity of norms and principles of justice that are drawn from a reservoir of value-consensus that exists prior to any public discourse. For the proceduralist, dialogue establishes the rules on which all conversation partners can agree. For contextualists, dialogue mediates what modern thought has differentiated—facts and values, rules and application, the right and the good, the individual and the community, form and content, methodological and substantive problems.

These distinctions yield different notions of what dialogue is. For contextualists, dialogue is conversation modelled on the intimate (face-to-face) dialogue of persons. Dialogue is the structure of interpersonal and intracontextual communication. It is the intersubjective framework of understanding, communicational action and consensus building as an arena of shared meaning, shared interpretations and shared action. What is shared is given by context, but it is also expanded by context. It develops, changes and is transformed by conversation. In this interpretive horizon, ethics is dominated by interpretation. Thus, contextualism grounds a theory of meaning rather than a theory of truth.

For proceduralists, dialogue is discourse as argumentation that offers clear, adequate reasons for one position over another, for one value over another, for one interpretation over another. Thus, attention is focussed on the conditions for communication rather than the act or even the structure of communicating. Procedural normativity is what is of paramount concern. Thus, proceduralism heads toward a theory of truth.[26]

Given these differences, it is not surprising then that there are different notions of what dialogue validates. For contextualists, validity is the social binding force of values, imperatives, rules and laws. A norm is valid when it is socially enacted and socially accepted. For proceduralists, validity is the rational legitimacy of the procedures that guarantee fairness of process and universal participation in public dialogue. Where liberals and critical theorists disagree is over the degree of institutional control required to assure impartiality and fairness.

This brings us to the real heart of this debate, which is about the relationship of "private" and "public" worlds. For contextualists, the private and public intersect as tradition—shared conversation about values, interests and meanings. Culture forms the individual even as individuals contribute to cultural patterns and understanding. Culture provides the form and content of personal identity and is a point of personal identification. Private values are literally absorbed from the public context of tradition and culture. Liberal and critical proceduralists, on the other hand, separate the private from the public, seeking to find a balance to assure the greatest personal freedom from public coercion. For liberals, this means the smallest public sphere possible in favour of an enlarged private sphere. For critical theorists, this means the desire to institutionalize the processes of critical reflection in a manner that assures optimal personal freedom. In all three cases, however, the public is a means to an end that yields an instrumental rationality that governs the public sphere. This is the critical problem at the heart of the private–public nexus that must be surmounted.

This debate, as it stands, highlights the issues that make moral affirmations difficult. Neither position is able to overcome the basic context-dependent/context-independent dichotomy that has given rise to the debate and which continues to drive it forward. The context-dependent position fails to develop an adequate notion of critical judgment that permits one to judge the rightness or wrongness within or among traditions. The context-independent position has a notion of judgment, but its notion of normative justification has difficulty rising above a circular argument with regard to the justification of foundational normative claims.

Context-dependent positions, such as MacIntyre's, are able to account for the sedimentation of normative experience in traditions, institutions,

---

26. On the difference between a theory of truth and a theory of meaning see, Richard Kirkham, *Theories of Truth: A Critical Introduction* (Cambridge: MIT Press, 1992), chap. 3.

language, history and the like, but they fail to account adequately for the sense of human freedom with regard to traditions and their values. Formalist positions, such as Habermas and Ackerman's, by starting with the problem of freedom, demonstrate the malleability of norms with regard to their human content, but fail to account adequately for the sense of givenness of social roles and social institutions as value sedimentations within human experience. So what we are left with is a two-headed notion that dialogue is a structure (norm) and yet transformative (malleable). But the question that is not answered is what is dialogue such that it is both normative and transformative and provides a link between private and public worlds?

PAUL RICOEUR AND THE CONVERSATION OF ETHICS

Paul Ricoeur is a philosopher in the hermeneutic tradition whose philosophical project has centred on understanding the connection between language and action. According to Ricoeur, language as communication is the locus for the articulation of experience. Experience supports language. Consequently everything does not arrive in language, but only comes to language. In turn, moral experience is Ricoeur's entry to the dialogical turn in ethics as he confronts the question "What is the human experience of normative action and value?"

To answer this question, Ricoeur starts with a notion of "ethical intentionality," which, he argues, precedes morality as law, norm or imperative. This intentionality consists of three interrelated experiences that move from the personal self to impersonal institutions or through the private to the public. The first experience is the experience of the self as free. Indeed, the self is realized in the effort to secure its liberty. This fundamental notion yields an ethic of action.

However, the self is not an atomistic free individual. The self also encounters, is contested by, the other who is also seeking to realize its freedom. That is, the self as "I" encounters the opposition of the liberty of the "second person," the other ("thou"), in the sphere of personal action. This is to say that one encounters the demands and imperatives of interaction. This relationship is a dialogical interaction of "willing the liberty of the second person." This is the dialogue of intimate relationship, of family, home and friendship. It is the dimension of "love" that spontaneously seeks the good of the other and has no need of "rules" or normative "justification." The ethic of the second person is the dimension of personal and interpersonal action that yields an ethics of interaction.

The third movement of ethical intentionality and the proper dimension of public dialogue is the experience of the impersonal "third person."

These are the larger social relationships of socially cooperative living, which are not bound by intimate relations, but impersonal relations guided by imperatives, rules and norms, that is, relationships that are not mediated by direct (face-to-face) conversational interaction, but by the rules and normative expectations of impersonal social intercourse.[27] Ricoeur characterizes this dimension of the socially impersonal as an ongoing conversation. Thus, the intimate self through the sociality of the impersonal human being, "enters into a conversation that precedes me, to which I contribute for a certain period of time, and that continues after me."[28] This is a conversation in which, "the ethical life is a perpetual transaction between the project of freedom and its ethical situation outlined by the given world of institutions."[29]

It is important to note that the ethical movement for Ricoeur is a move from self to institutions through value to imperative and law.[30] This movement is one from the sphere of the intimately personal to the objectively impersonal, from the intimately known to the anonymous. This movement from the intimate self to impersonal other requires a greater and greater specification of the acceptable reasons for actions, a greater formalism and a higher level of normative justification. This model of discourse frames three significant clarifications to the relationship of the private and public spheres of value as they are mediated by dialogue.

First, ethical discourse is open to experience and experience to explanation. There is a reciprocal relationship between morality as social praxis and ethics as a critical justification of acts according to law, principles or theory.

Ricoeur's three-step model shows precisely what is different between the private and public spheres, but also shows why the private sphere

---

27. A simple example of the difference between the private and public spheres is provided by my desire (a personal desire) to get home this afternoon. In driving home I have neither the desire nor the interest in personally negotiating (intimate dialogue) the rules of the road that will allow me to drive my car from the university to my home. The driving code (which consists of the code and the requisite skills to perform the complex transactions implicit in the code) permits a set of mutual (and impersonal) expectations to come into being without having on each occasion of driving my car to bring such normative expectations into being. The impersonal scheme is dynamized originally by a personal desire, but the operation of the scheme that operates independently of my desire does not require my personal dialogic approval or disapproval of the scheme. The scheme is the condition of the possibility of my being able to drive safely. This is to say that in willing a result or state of affairs, I must also will the conditions of the result. The scheme, not my desires, provides the normative structure, as articulated in imperative, rules, laws and principles.

28. Ricoeur, "Avant la loi morale," 43b.

29. Ricoeur, "Ethics and Culture," 269.

30. Ricoeur, "Avant la loi morale," 45a.

necessarily moves to the public. The architecture of the self includes a public dimension. Liberal-critical proceduralism tries to preserve a critical and real distinction that is essential to human freedom, but the distinction is purchased at the price of misunderstanding what is at stake in the private-public differentiation and so isolates the private from the public with the concomitant necessity of trying to bridge artificially what is really immanent in human experience. Communitarians, on the other hand, will not tolerate a private–public distinction. They preserve the private sphere of the self, but at the price of undervaluing the necessary formalism of the public action.

Second, there is a difference between dialogue as intimate conversation in reciprocal reflexive understanding and discourse as a public process of offering adequate reasons for normative action or understanding.[31] One can reasonably assume that intimate dialogue, the ethic of intimate interaction, does resolve value conflicts and disagreements about values, principles and norms of action. There is no reason to assume that public dialogue as a process of argumentation and justification ought to be able to accomplish the same thing when it is recognized that the intelligibility of procedures is the facilitation of the value of social relationships. Indeed, rules of discourse are required in order to assure reasonable disagreement about norms and values in a public forum.[32] But such rules permanently contest an imperial self that tries to impose itself in its liberty. Such contestation yields the "true self" that is known in its relations. That is, the structural requirements that sustain schemes of public discourse operate to shift and transform the values dynamizing the intimate self as the self interacts through such schemes.

This insight drives to the heart of the liberal misconception of value. Liberals argue that one cannot have a public discussion about values because values represent some non-negotiable architecture of the self. But they define value *a priori* in a way that will not allow values into the public sphere. Communitarians understand that values drive social interaction forward and so conflicts about values are not pathological, but genuinely creative. What communitarians fail to appreciate adequately, however, is how public values can become systematically distorted and require the critical judgment of reason.

---

31. Ricoeur, "Hermeneutics and the Critique of Ideology," 91-92: "in contrast to the simple discourse of conversation, which enters into the spontaneous movement of question and answer, discourse as a work 'takes hold' in structures calling for a description and an explanation that mediate 'understanding.'"

32. If anyone has ever watched children playing a game, an action that embodies characteristics of both intimate interaction and public formalism, one has an excellent example of how discourse about rules resolves conflicts about rules to permit greater freedom of intimate action.

Third, an ethics of personal relationship is more intimately related to the realm of desire, that is, personal value, than public discourse, which is related to the impersonal dimension of social institutions and justice.[33] The normative dynamism that governs institutions is related directly to the realm of (social, public) order[34] and its legitimation, which is ultimately historically conditioned.[35] However, as Ricoeur argues, the fact that the law legitimates a public order giving personal desires, values and norms the "stamp" of universal accord does not mean that the order is free of criticism. Indeed, what is required is that one return to reconsider the concrete actions that fulfil the criterion of the law. This is to acknowledge that as discourse has a normative structure to it that makes certain requirements on anyone who joins the conversation, any sphere of human living will have a structure that imposes requirements whose procedures make normative demands on contents.

WHAT CAN WE LEARN?

What do we learn from this talk about talk? First, the realm of value is fundamentally social. While the starting point of morality is the first person (an intentional "I"), the ethical imperative arises in or through an experience of contestation or opposition. Conflicts of values are interpersonal and intersubjective, and discourse or dialogue is the vehicle of opposition (i.e., the experience of conflict "comes" to language). However, the socio-cooperative project of civilization and civilizing extends beyond any intimate "I-Thou" relationship to include the dimension of the impersonal other. That is, ethics is a product of sociability, and sociability is constituted by a complex recurrent scheme of communication. This means dialogue exhibits two movements with regard to value and normativity: the element of the personal, the individual who intends, desires, wants and needs; and the ineluctably cooperative schemes of social interaction.

Second, the public–private distinction cannot be reasonably sustained. The complex interrelationship of sociability is not a simply "individual–collective" (private–public, person–institutional) dichotomy, but a complex human transaction of individuals socio-cooperatively linked by recurrent schemes of interaction of which language structured as conversation is the most complex. Language is not simply a vehicle of "self–other"

---

33. Paul Ricoeur, "Le juste entre le bon et le légal," *Esprit* (September 1991).

34. Ricoeur, "Avant la loi morale," 45b.

35. Ricoeur, "Hermeneutics and the Critique of Ideology," 76-78.

interaction, it is also the tool of all conscious thought. Language is the link between private and public worlds.[36]

Third, a complete understanding of what dialogue accomplishes can methodologically correct our assumptions about public discourse. The complex scheme of social interaction is not a simple either/or choice between the private and public sphere. If this were true, language and communication would be impossible. If we are attentive to experience, we recognize that language, talking, dialogue and discourse do create possibilities and potentials for changes of values, judgments of value and new courses of normative action that do in fact occur in the dialogical situation where significant values are at stake.

The essential point is, I think, discourse does mediate values to a significant degree. What we need to be sure of when we talk about values is what level or dimension of value is in play, what kind of value dissensus is moving a particular conflict forward and what kind of consensus is the anticipated outcome of talking.[37] Frankly, it seems human beings have three options open in conflicted situations: they can fight to impose a solution, they can withdraw from interaction or they can talk it out. A viable human project is one that takes the third option seriously in spite of its risks and problems or our lack of theoretical understanding of what happens when we agree to talk.

---

36. A complete justification of this claim is beyond the competence of this chapter. However, see the argument developed by Stuart Hampshire in *Thought and Action* with which I am in essential agreement. However, Hampshire's application of this work to ethics in *Morality and Conflict* does not carry through on the promises of his theory of intentional action as developed in *Thought and Action*.

37. See James B. Sauer, "Values, Transactions, and Consensus," May 1992, TMs [photocopy], Saint Paul University Centre for Techno-Ethics, Ottawa.

Chapter 7

The Cognitional Theory of Bernard Lonergan and the Structure of Ethical Deliberation

Kenneth R. Melchin

The preceding chapter by James Sauer presents a brief overview and analysis of some of the principal contributors to the theoretical literature in discourse ethics. Sauer identifies two main approaches in this literature, the contextualists and the proceduralists.

The focus of the proceduralists (e.g., Habermas, Rawls, Ackerman) is on the structure of ethical discourse and/or the political contracts and institutions that establish procedures for adjudicating conflicting value claims. Their interest is in general structural features that operate in all ethical discourse regardless of context or ethical content. In their view, all participants are rationally bound to accept these norms or obligations whenever they seek to advance their ethical claims through discourse.

The focus of the contextualists (e.g., Gadamer, MacIntyre, Sandel) is on the social, cultural, historical traditions and contexts of meaning that inform ethical claims, and which set the framework for adjudicating among conflicting claims. Foundational norms or principles for resolving ethical disputes are to be found in the analysis of cultural contexts of ethical meaning, which the parties implicitly draw upon in advancing their claims. The contextualists argue that purely formal or discourse-structure approaches themselves draw upon traditions for their notions of obligation and rationality and that a full grounding of their own theories requires appropriating these traditions.

Sauer's chapter draws upon the work of Paul Ricoeur to argue that these two theoretical approaches do not present mutually exclusive analyses of ethical discourse. Rather, they highlight two realms of normativity operative in ethical discourse that interact to drive the dynamics of discourse in complex dialectical ways. To understand what is going on in discourse requires analyzing both the interpersonal contexts of moral meaning operative in the discourse as well as procedural aspects of the discourse structure.

While Sauer's analysis does not put an end to the debates in discourse ethics, it does provide grounds for a direction where a synthesis might be found. If these two theoretical approaches do not offer conflicting analyses of the same phenomena but complementary analyses of distinct realms of normativity operative in the ethical discourse, then it would seem to make sense to analyze discourse in both realms. These two realms would need to be reflected in formulating practical guides for ethical discourse in health care teams.

Sauer's argument for the complementarity of these two approaches is based in Ricoeur's analysis of a structured "intentionality" operative in linguistic meaning. Bernard Lonergan has developed a theory of human cognition that offers a comprehensive explanation of "intentionality" as it operates in diverse realms of meaning and patterns of human experience. Because it is based in an empirical analysis of operations of human cognition as they function in all activities of human knowing and valuing, Lonergan's theory suggests itself as a framework for carrying forward the insights of Ricoeur and integrating the contributions from various fields of research in ethics. In addition, Lonergan's work offers grounds for understanding how various individuals' operations of meaning can group together to form structures of sociality that can function quite apart from the planning or explicit understanding of any individuals.[1] Consequently, this framework promises insights that may help link the respective concerns for the personal and the public realms of value of the contextualists and the proceduralists.

The strategy in this chapter will be to set out Lonergan's fourfold structure of cognition as a framework for responding to the concerns of the proceduralists and the contextualists and to explore some implications for ethical discourse in health care teams.

THE FOURFOLD STRUCTURE OF COGNITION

Lonergan's philosophy is based upon four distinct levels of operations that are involved in human cognition.[2] While Lonergan developed his fourfold structure in the study of cognition as operative in scientific

---

1. See, for example, Kenneth R. Melchin, *History, Ethics, and Emergent Probability* (Lanham, Md.: University Press of America, 1987); Patrick H. Byrne, "Jane Jacobs and the Common Good," in *Ethics in Making a Living*, ed. Fred Lawrence (Atlanta: Scholars Press, 1989), 169-189; Philip McShane, *Randomness, Statistics and Emergence* (Dublin: Gill and Macmillan, 1970).

2. See Bernard Lonergan, *Method*, chap. 1, for a summary presentation of the four levels of cognitional operations.

understanding, his own work and that of others has carried this forward into a theory of ethics.[3]

Lonergan's work has been described as a generalized empirical method. It is empirical insofar as the insights into cognitional operations are not based upon philosophical speculation or logical analysis but upon any human subject's empirical attention to his or her own acts of cognition as they occur in the process of understanding something.[4] While the method involves a scrutiny of personal cognitional operations, the results of this scrutiny are fully public insofar as all persons can appeal to a similar database and, as with all sciences, conflicting results can result in critical dialogue among scholars that refines theories and corrects errors. While this method does not appeal to the same types of laboratory or statistical controls as are found in the natural or social sciences, still Lonergan has developed canons of method that subject hypotheses to rigorous scrutiny in the operations of verification.[5] Lonergan's claim to the generality of this method is based upon the empirical argument that any person who would refute his insights into cognitional operations would have to use them in the refutation.[6]

---

3. For an introduction to the secondary literature in Lonergan's ethics, see the following: Joseph P. Cassidy, *Extending Bernard Lonergan's Ethics*, Ph.D. dissertation, Saint Paul University, Ottawa, 1995; Michael Vertin, "Judgments of Value for the Later Lonergan," *Method: Journal of Lonergan Studies* 13 (Fall 1995): 221-248; Kenneth R. Melchin, *Living with Other People* (Ottawa: Novalis/Collegeville: Liturgical Press, 1998); Kenneth R. Melchin, "Pluralism, Conflict, and the Structure of the Public Good," in *The Promise of Critical Theology*, ed. Marc Lalonde (Waterloo: Wilfred Laurier University Press, 1995): 75-92; Kenneth R. Melchin, "Economics, Ethics, and the Structure of Social Living," *Humanomics* 10, no. 3 (1994): 21-57; Kenneth R. Melchin, "Moral Knowledge and the Structure of Cooperative Living," *Theological Studies* 52 (September 1991): 495-523; Patrick H. Byrne, "'Ressentiment' and the Preferential Option for the Poor," *Theological Studies* 54 (1993): 214-241; Cynthia Crysdale, "Revisioning Natural Law: From the Classicist Paradigm to Emergent Probability," *Theological Studies* 56 (1995): 464-484; Fred Lawrence, "The Fragility of Consciousness: Lonergan and the Postmodern Concern for the Other," *Theological Studies* 54 (1993): 55-94; Stephen Happel and James J. Walter, *Conversion and Discipleship* (Philadelphia: Fortress Press, 1986); Walter E. Conn, *Conversion: Development and Self-Transcendence* (Birmingham, Al.: Religious Education Press, 1981); Frederick Crowe, "An Exploration of Lonergan's New Notion of Value," *Science et Esprit* 29 (1977): 123-143; Frederick Crowe, "An Expansion of Lonergan's Notion of Value," in *Lonergan Workshop*, ed. Fred Lawrence (Atlanta: Scholars Press, 1988), 35-57; Philip McShane, *Wealth of Self and Wealth of Nations* (Hicksville, N.Y.: Exposition Press, 1975).

4. The empirical base for this work is developed in *Insight*.

5. For the canons of empirical method, see *Insight*, chap. 3.

6. See *Method*, 19-20, for the presentation of this argument.

Lonergan describes the four levels of cognitional operations as experience, understanding, judgment and decision. In any type of inquiry, the first level is *experience*, which presents perceptions, hunches, notions, data to be examined and feelings to be explored. The move to the second level, to the operations of *understanding*, takes the materials of experience and views them in the light of specific questions. In the effort to understand things, we stop taking them for granted and start examining them, probing them, looking for new aspects. The driving force of understanding is the question and the product is the insight, which grasps an intelligibility in the data of experience that claims to answer the question. However, insights often yield partial, incomplete, misleading or wrong answers. Consequently, the third level involves *judgment*, the critical scrutiny of our insights in search of a more comprehensive understanding that satisfies the demands of our inquiring. Here, we want to know if the insights stand the test of our questions and our experiences. When we find holes in our insights, when we find them partial, when we find them problematic, we go back to experience in search of clues for new insights. When judgment proclaims the full set of insights to stand up to our collective questioning, then we move on to the fourth level of *decision* and action. This level involves putting things into practice, it involves acting in the light of our knowledge, it calls for integrity and honesty.

The fourth level of decision involves the sorts of things that we commonly associate with ethics. However, ethicists working with Lonergan's theories have shown how all four levels of cognitional operations function both in the realms of factual knowledge and ethical knowledge.[7] Ethics does not only involve acting on known values, it involves the entire process of experiencing, understanding and judging wherein we come to know values. Consequently, when the four levels of cognitional operations are turned to ethical inquiry, the goals or objects of all four levels of operations take on a distinctive ethical character.

---

7. For discussions of the distinctive character of the operations in the realm of ethical knowledge, see the works of Cassidy, *Extending Bernard Lonergan's Ethics*; McShane, *Wealth of Self and Wealth of Nations*; Melchin, "Economics, Ethics, and the Structure of Social Living" and "Moral Knowledge and the Structure of Cooperative Living."

FOUR LEVELS OF ETHICAL MEANING

When the inquiry is ethical, the four levels of cognitional operations have the effect of transforming the meaning of ethical language.[8] Values as experienced in feelings of desire have a different structure of meaning than values as understood, and judged, for example, as the codes of conduct of professional practice. Both are ethical or moral, both involve feelings and desires, and both have implications for action.[9] However, the structure of meaning of the two are quite different. Furthermore, an analysis of these differences, we suggest, can set the stage for understanding the complementary contributions of the proceduralist and contextualist theories of discourse ethics.

On the first level of cognitional operations, the level of experience, ethical value is experienced as the object of our immediate, practical desire or *interest*.[10] Here, the good is usually stated as what we want, as a straightforward position that we wish to pursue. In public discourse, ethical language on this level of meaning yields diverse desires, objectives and positions. Here is where ethical diversity and conflict first appear, for, as we all know, desires are multiple and conflicting.

On the second level of understanding, ethical language comes to mean something different. Here, we cease taking our immediate practical interests for granted as the last word. In understanding, we begin questioning, probing, looking for ethical insights. Our search is for reasons why we want what we want and we find answers through understanding social

---

8. In *Insight*, Lonergan presents the structure of the good as having three levels; see chap. 18. However, between *Insight* and *Method*, Lonergan developed a fourth level; see Crowe, "An Exploration." The presentation of the fourth level is taken up in *Method*, in the discussion of the structure of the human good, in chap. 2, 47-52. My presentation, which is developed in the following pages, is a simplified account of how the four levels of cognitional operations yield four different levels of ethical meaning. As is clear from a study of Lonergan's texts, his understanding is somewhat more complex. However, I would argue that the essentials are retained.

9. While many ethicists make a distinction between the meanings of the terms "ethical" and "moral," no distinction is implied here.

10. I have not followed Lonergan's terms in presenting the four levels of ethical meaning. In *Insight*, chap. 18, Lonergan uses the terms "desire," "good of order" and "value" for the first three levels. In *Method*, chap. 2, he uses the terms "particular good," "good of order" and "terminal value," and speaks of the cognitional level of "decision," which renders a transformation in the intentional thrust of the previous three to yield their distinctive objects when governed by the intentionality of decision and action. I have chosen the terms "interest," "social order," "evaluation" and "action" in an effort to capture a language that might be more accessible to practitioners in health care. I would argue that I have retained the central thrust of Lonergan's meaning in this presentation.

relations. The good or the right on this second level is understood as *social order*. Ethical value here refers to the obligations and goals associated with the institutions and relationships that enable the fulfilment of wide ranges of desires of all participants in society.

What is interesting about this second level of value is that our understanding of social relationships often comes to light through probing our feelings. While some feelings express little more than personal desires or interests, other feelings often point beyond mere interest toward more complex social values to which we are drawn but that lie hidden to us. Feelings often move us ethically without revealing the values that are their objects.[11] It is in probing these feelings, in seeking to understanding the social relationships that they intend, that we can effect the transition from the level of interest to the level of social order.

Whether these relations of social order are local (e.g., familial or interpersonal) or more general (e.g., professional or legal) still the object of this second level of ethical understanding pertains to the values, obligations and goals associated with schemes of social order. This is the level of codes of ethical conduct. It is also the level of implicit ethical obligations that arise in connection with professions, institutions and other forms of emergent social order.

The third level of ethical meaning arises when we discover that ethical understanding can be incomplete, mistaken or deliberately distorted and that social orders can be flawed, corrupt or oppressive. At this point our concerns and questions shift to the operations of ethical deliberation, where we sort out true values from false values. Our goal here is the judgment or ethical *evaluation*. Here, our task is to distinguish between notions of social order and obligation that are truly good and those that are unjust or oppressive. To do so, ethics must seek to understand social orders within the wider contexts of historical or ecological process and ask whether social orders are agents of progress or decline. Currently, such things as charters of rights and international codes of conduct are efforts to express this third level of ethical value. However, great literature, art and drama, as well as significant historical works, also function on this level of evaluation.[12]

---

11. On feelings as intentional responses to values, see Lonergan, *Method*, 30-34. There are remarkable similarities between this presentation and Cheryl Picard's account of the role of the exploration of feelings in conflict mediation. See Cheryl A. Picard, *Mediating Interpersonal and Small Group Conflict* (Ottawa: Golden Dog Press, 1998). Picard does not refer to the underlying concerns revealed in feelings as values. However, in the following chapter by Peter Monette, the role of values in conflicts is discussed.

12. See, for example, David Tracy, *The Analogical Imagination: Christian Theology and the Culture of Pluralism* (New York: Crossroads, 1986), and Gibson Winter, *Liberating Creation* (New York: Crossroads, 1981).

The operations of ethical evaluation can only be carried out in a fully public ethical discourse. This is because evaluation requires examining social orders in the light of the experiences of all people who are implicated in their operation. Carrying out this task of evaluation involves consulting the experiences of all stakeholders. While traditional ethical theories often envision this third level of value as a set of universal principles binding on all people at all times, Lonergan understands the third level of value dynamically or historically. Human societies never stand outside of history; rather, we are always seeking to understand the directions of justice and progress from within history. Consequently, we are continually in the process of discerning, evaluating and reevaluating the social orders that constitute our living. A continual, wide-scale reflection on history can give rise to later generations building on the insights and correcting the errors of earlier ages. Consequently, this third level of value continually involves a wide-scale public discourse that reflects on extant orders of social living and subjects them to critical scrutiny.[13]

The fourth level of cognitional operations involves commitment, decision and action. Here, ethical language refers to the practical programs of *action* that are formulated to implement the results of the deliberations. Decision requires more than an affirmation of value—it requires a commitment to action at specific times with specific divisions of labour. Action may be agreed to informally, but it may also be articulated in formal contracts and agreements that are mutually recognized as binding. In either case, what distinguishes this level of value are its specific obligations for implementation.

Lonergan describes the cognitional operations as levels. This implies a vertical or hierarchical ordering rather than a horizontal or complementary ordering. The reason for this is that each level involves a set of operations of meaning and each level operates on the products of the previous levels, subjecting them to higher-level scrutiny and evaluating them within wider frames of reference. However, unlike other types of hierarchies, the higher levels do not render the lower levels obsolete or pronounce them immature or irrelevant. Rather, the higher levels take up the products of the lower-level operations and refine them so that we can return them to daily practice with greater care and precision. Interests and desires can be experienced and immediately acted upon. But they can also be probed and questioned, their objects understood and their goals

---

13. Lonergan did not explicitly present the operation of judgment of value in terms of public discourse. See *Method*, 36-41. However, his discussion of the functional special "dialectic," which operates on the fourth level of intentionality, the level of value, involves considerable public discourse. We begin to see some traces of how Lonergan foresaw the public discourse on value unfolding in dialectic in *Method*, chap. 10, particularly 247-249 and 253-257.

and implied obligations evaluated so that our decisions and actions are more careful, more responsible. When this occurs, ethical feelings can reveal the social relations that are their objects and thus be rendered all the more potent for responsible daily living.

The significance of this understanding of hierarchy becomes clearer when we begin asking about the relationship between the first and second levels of ethical value, interests and social order. The fact is that social living involves a vast array of complex, concretely functioning structures and institutions of social cooperation. Some of these have been planned. But many have emerged spontaneously in society and history. Examples of cooperation can be found everywhere: pushing a car out of a ditch, maintaining an automobile or a flower garden, building a house, doing research, raising children, designing and manufacturing computers, running a university, ensuring public security and governing a country.[14] In each case, results are achieved through the coordination of the diverse contributions of numbers of people toward a common purpose.

One of the most interesting aspects of cooperative schemes concerns the diversity of personal desires and interests that participants realize through the cooperative schemes. There seems to be no end to the variety of reasons why people cooperate with each other. While economic schemes, educational schemes, family schemes and health care schemes all have distinct objectives of their own, the range of particular interests that individuals seem to pursue in these schemes appears endless.

However, there is a marked difference between these diverse individual interests and the much narrower range of social objectives or requirements that arise from the structure of cooperation itself. Every effort of human cooperation involves participants submitting to specific demands that are set by the structure of the cooperative scheme. In businesses, employees must follow the routines of the business as well as the codes of the profession and the laws of the land in order for the work of the business to get done. In schools, curricula must be planned in the light of ordered programs of student development, and teachers must teach with sufficient skill and integrity for students to develop the insights and skills. In hospitals, the contributions of various professionals must be coordinated into responsible programs of patient care. And in all three spheres, participants need discourse skills, problem-solving skills and team-building skills to handle the hosts of interpersonal and job-related difficulties that arise through the course of a working day.

It is in analyzing the structure of social schemes that we come to understand the obligations that are entailed in their operation. Ethical

---

14. For analyses of emergent schemes and how they ground obligations, see Melchin, "Economics," "Moral Knowledge" and "Pluralism," and Byrne, "Jane Jacobs."

obligations like honesty, diligence, fair dealing and respect for patients and clients do not have their foundations in purely formal logical principles or abstract codes. They are rooted in the structure of social schemes as the requirements necessary for participants to maintain the schemes and the goods they make possible. Lonergan's concern with the good of order is not an abstract preoccupation with order. Rather, it is rooted in the understanding that social orders are the conduits through which all the elements of social living are delivered to society and that these conduits are complex schemes of social meaning that place obligations on the shoulders of all.

These ethical obligations of social order must take precedence over individual interests when the two conflict.[15] The fact is that personal desires can only be fulfilled through cooperative social living and structures of social cooperation can only harness the involvement of all if they aim at meeting not simply my desires but those of all contributors. Furthermore, social structures make their own demands on all who are implicated in their routines. Consequently, to live fully in society requires a willingness to accept the higher-level obligations rooted in the structure of social cooperation when they conflict with personal interests. This hierarchical relationship does not rule out personal interests. Quite the contrary. Social goods can also be the objects of personal interest and desire. In fact, a sustained commitment to social obligations can give rise to a transformation in personal habits of desiring. The hierarchical relationship between personal interest and social order does not abrogate desire; it understands the objects of desire by setting them within their wider context of social relations.

The hierarchical ordering of the levels of ethical meaning applies equally to the relationship between the second and third levels of value. Just as personal interest must submit to the understanding of social order, so too must social order submit to the judgment of communal, historical evaluation. When social structures and institutional routines begin to function as agents of oppression or ecological degradation, or when they begin to undermine fundamental conditions of equality and dignity of peoples, they must submit to ethical critique. Ethical evaluation recognizes social order but not at any price. When placed within the wider contexts

---

15. Patrick Byrne refers to this type of ethical theory as a "common good" theory. However, he discusses the difference between classicist and dynamic notions of the "common good." There are notable similarities between this understanding of the normative priority of social values and that of Daly and Cobb in Herman Daly and John B. Cobb, Jr., *For the Common Good* (Boston: Beacon Press, 1989). For a similar type of analysis that appeals to the structure of spheres of social order to ground an understanding of justice, see Michael Walzer, *Spheres of Justice* (New York: Basic Books, 1983).

of world society, history and ecological process, social orders can be understood either as agents of progress or of injustice and decline. This critical, evaluative work is the task of judgment. And judgment accomplishes its task through the wide-scale public discourse that consults the experiences and understandings of all citizens.

As with the second level, the third level of ethical meaning is not a matter of purely logical principles or abstract codes. Rather, the work of judgment is the public effort of discourse that scrutinizes structures of social order wherever they operate, assesses their operation within the wider ecologies of social relations that constitute the world environment, discerns the patterns of transformation that their functioning is effecting in relation to past and future social realities and potentialities, and evaluates this direction of transformation as progress or decline. Because our knowledge of historical value is always achieved within history, our notions of progress and decline will develop and unfold as we encounter new moments in world process and as wider circles of citizens gain entry into the public discourse of historical valuation. Consequently, one of the fundamental requirements of this discourse is the full participation of all.

Currently, the discourse of historical evaluation is unfolding in the language of such things as universal human rights, world war crimes tribunals and declarations of environmental obligations. These notions arise out of dramatic experiences of decline like the Holocaust and the prognoses of global ecological disaster. They seek to counter decline by articulating basic obligatory features of social order that all peoples must recognize if our social living is to avoid catastrophe. Judgments of evaluation do not abrogate social order. Rather, they set the conditions and requirements that social orders must meet.

Finally, the fourth level of ethical meaning, the level of action, imposes its own requirements on judgments of value. Values must not only be affirmed as true, they must also be put into action. When the demands of action are faced concretely, what comes to light is the difference between abstract speculation and real possibilities. To implement values requires implementing them in real life and real life is fraught with limitations and contradictions. Consequently, the demands of action require facing the social situation as it is and making the commitment to move things forward from this point. This requires assessing ranges of possibilities and limitations as well obligations and responsibilities.

The four levels of ethical meaning do not dictate any concrete principles that are immediately applicable to ethical situations. Rather, they provide a map of the full set of operations that are involved in ethical discourse and they can furnish indications of the kinds of transformations in ethical meaning that arise when we move from one level of operations to another. In the next section, we will explore the potentialities of this theoretical framework for locating and assessing the contributions of various theorists to a comprehensive understanding of ethical discourse.

PROCEDURALISTS, CONTEXTUALISTS AND THE STRUCTURE OF ETHICAL MEANING

What becomes clear from Sauer's analysis of the proceduralist and contextualist theories of ethical discourse is that both lines of theory seek to develop criteria for judgments of ethical evaluation. Both offer frameworks for critically evaluating social processes and, consequently, both function on Lonergan's third level of ethical meaning. However, what is interesting is that neither proceduralists nor contextualists differentiate among the multiple levels of ethical meaning. The effect is that theorists from the two approaches tend to regard ethics quite differently, depending on which level of meaning they take to be the language of ethics. Furthermore, both the proceduralists and the contextualists appeal to very specific realms of social structures to establish their framework for evaluation and judgment. For the proceduralist, the normative structures are to be found in the analysis of the institutions and procedures of discourse itself. For the contextualist, the normative social structures are those of the cultural tradition whose context of meaning sets the framework for interpreting the content of ethical claims.

In the view of liberal theorists like Rawls and Ackerman, ethics is understood in terms of the distinction between the realms of the public and the private. The private is the realm of individual opinion and interest, the realm where an irreducible plurality of moral views must be respected. This is the realm of ethics and ethics is simply a matter of individual desire, interest, opinion—Lonergan's first level of ethical meaning. This private sphere of individual interest can make no claim on the public sphere, nor can a probing of interests or desires be expected to reveal their rational grounding in structures of social order. The public sphere must be reserved only for those principles, procedures and institutions that guarantee individual liberties and regulate individuals' interest claims.

While Habermas does not confine the meaning of the term "ethics" exclusively to the level of personal interest, he does share Rawls' and Ackerman's convictions about the irreducible plurality of values. Furthermore, he shares their view that public discourse cannot evaluate and pronounce on the content of value claims. Consequently, he turns to an analysis of the structure of discourse for his criteria for regulating value disputes. Habermas does allow the term "ethics" to apply to this social discourse activity. However, like the liberal theorists, he does not recognize this as a higher level of ethical meaning because he does not recognize multiple levels of ethical meaning. Consequently, public discourse cannot pronounce on the content of value claims—it can only establish a range of procedures whereby participants in discourse can live with irreducible value differences.

The communitarians, on the other hand, recognize that value conflicts often can be resolved by appealing to the wider contexts of meaning of cultural traditions. In fact, for MacIntyre, the goal of ethics is to evaluate value claims against this backdrop of culture and tradition. This is clearly Lonergan's third level of ethical meaning. However, communitarians do not differentiate the second from the third levels of ethical operations. Consequently, value judgments are judgments of coherence within traditions. They do not recognize that an understanding of social structures and ecologies of structures could yield ethical criteria for critically evaluating the tradition, criteria that may not be gleaned from a tradition's own self-articulation.

What communitarians do recognize is that individual interests and desires (the first level of ethical meaning) can be evaluated critically in public discourse. Contrary to the proceduralists, they see this happening all the time and recognize that such critical reflection on the content of personal interest is, in fact, the goal of public discourse. What they also recognize is that discourse structures only constitute one of the many realms of social structure whose analysis can yield norms for ethical evaluation. However, what they can learn from proceduralists is how the analysis of social structure can ground ethical evaluation and, indeed, how their own project of critical reflection on cultural traditions can be enhanced by the careful analysis of the variety of social structures that make up the tradition.

Finally, what Lonergan's analysis can offer both lines of theory is an understanding of the full range of operations and levels of meaning in ethical discourse. Proceduralists who despair of the possibility of a public consensus on values take the first level of ethical meaning, the level of desire, to be the only level of ethical meaning. By moving through the operations on the second, third and fourth levels, public ethical discourse can locate and critically evaluate the foundations and contexts of our desires and interests. The public character of our common participation in the full range of social structures and institutions furnishes both a need and a ground for a public ethical discourse. A need, because cooperative schemes require a significant measure of agreement on the part of all participants if they are to continue functioning. And a ground, because the diverse perspectives of all participants on this common experience can shed light on the multiple dimensions of a common social reality. Ethical discourse can aim at consulting these diverse views toward a more complete understanding of the responsibilities that flow from cooperative living.

CONFLICT AND ETHICAL DELIBERATION IN HEALTH CARE TEAMS

The cognitional theory of Bernard Lonergan suggests an ethical theory framework for understanding the respective contributions of the contextualist and proceduralist theories of ethical discourse. While both approaches seek an evaluative framework for assessing and adjudicating conflicting value claims, they do so by appealing to different spheres of social structures that are implicated in ethical discourse. The communitarians recognize that participants in discourse advance their value claims within cultural contexts of meaning and an analysis of the meaning structures common to both parties can yield criteria that both would have to accept as binding. The proceduralists recognize that discourse is a social structure of its own whose analysis can yield norms and obligations that are binding upon all who would seek to achieve their goals through discourse.

Both lines of theory can be enhanced by an appreciation of the levels of operations of ethical cognition. Both can benefit from an understanding of the diversity of realms of social structures that will yield diverse and conflicting norms and obligations. Furthermore, both would be enhanced by an appreciation of how the four levels of operations can be implemented to help participants work through these realms of conflict in ethical deliberation. Lonergan's theory does not provide immediate solutions to concrete ethical issues in health care. Ethical deliberation in concrete cases still requires the communitarian and proceduralist lines of analysis. However, the levels of ethical meaning represent four stages of operations that participants in health care teams must pass through in their ethical deliberations. Lonergan's theory can provide insights into how these operations unfold and how they effect transformations in the concrete value claims. While a full analysis of the dynamics of these operations in diverse fields of ethical discourse would far exceed the resources and aims of this research project, an initial sketch can provide a direction for research in the third stage of the project.

Ethical deliberation begins with the articulation of the interests of all parties in the discourse. The first level of operations requires that the full range of interests relevant to the case be articulated. For this to happen, all relevant parties must have full, unconstrained input into the discourse. Most often, the result of this first round of input is a diverse set of interests or positions articulated by the various members of the deliberation team. When this diversity is easily reconciled to the satisfaction of all parties, the following stages are straightforward. However, when this does not happen, ethical discourse must move beyond the level of interests to the exploration of the deeper levels of ethical meaning that are implicated in the interests.

The second level of operations involves a probing of these interests to identify the social structures that are implicated in the deliberation. Here is where the respective contributions of the communitarian and proceduralist lines of analysis come in. Probing the interests articulated by the interlocutors will reveal diverse ranges of social relations and structures that affect the case. Some of these structures will be those of the health care institutions and of the professionals implicated in the care delivery. Other relevant structures will be the family, religious, community and cultural relationships that define the life context of the patients and clients under care. Both of these realms will call for the communitarian lines of analysis. However, there is a third realm of structure, the structure of the discourse itself. This is the realm for proceduralist analysis and this includes the structures involved in the institutional forms of discourse as well as the structures that unfold in the resolution of conflicts. A full understanding of the interests operative in the discourse will usually require attention to all of these realms of social structure.

In order to move through the third level of ethical deliberation, the level of evaluation, participants in the discourse need some reflective awareness of how they are being motivated and directed by one, then another, of these realms of value. Guided by the norms governing the procedures of discourse, the participants need to probe the various realms of social structures and relations to identify the driving concerns of all. This requires the entire team engaging in a deliberate effort to appreciate the various realms of value that are the concerns of all the parties. The foundations for collective evaluation will be found in the common grounds that unite them all in discourse and which specify the common objectives of the program of care. When this is identified, the common grounds provide criteria for evaluating and prioritizing the other value claims in the case.

The fourth level of operations, the level of action, requires assessing the common objectives with an eye to practical implementation. Common values must be translated into action strategies and action strategies must be possible within real life institutional contexts. In addition, action strategies involve divisions of labour and tasks must be possible within the life and work routines of all team members if they are to be realized. Finally, proposed strategies must be put into real life practice, and this involves commitment. This final stage of operations involves scrutinizing common goals with these concerns in mind.

In this project, the documentary analysis of part 1, the implicit ethics of health care professionals, whose results are presented in the chapters by Jean-Marc Larouche and Tim Flaherty, represents a contextualist approach to ethical discourse. The normativity of the ethical claims of the various professionals is grounded in the specific context of meaning operative in the implicit self-understanding of each professional type. Furthermore, the dynamic interactions among the various professionals arise not from general features of discourse itself but from the specific conflicts and complementarities among the meaning contexts of the professional types.

In order for health care teams to deal effectively with ethical conflicts, professionals need to understand the implicit ethical claims of their own professional types and recognize the same in others. Furthermore, in situations of conflict, they need to move beyond the limitations of these contexts and strive to find common ethical horizons. The contextualist analysis would suggest that such common horizons are to be found in an understanding of the wider social and institutional contexts that set the common environment for their professional interaction. However, this analysis must also recognize the obligations that flow from the structure of discourse itself. This requires turning to proceduralist analyses of discourse.

The following chapter by Peter Monette summarizes the results of research in the field of conflict resolution and represents a proceduralist approach to ethical discourse. Conflict analysts and practitioners are not directly concerned with the cultural or professional contexts of meaning of the value claims of the parties in the discourse. Rather, their concern is to identify and rectify structural dysfunctions in the discourse process that exacerbate conflicts and present barriers to the exploration of common horizons of meaning and value. The analysis of the stages of conflictual discourse yields common procedural norms for guiding the parties through the stages of the discourse toward resolution. The analysis of discourse skills yields tools that can help the parties through this process.

Contrary to the expectations of contextualist and proceduralist theorists, neither of these bodies of theory on their own will yield complete sets of principles for the resolution of all aspects of value conflicts. Rather, value conflicts are only resolved by communities of men and women implementing the cognitional operations and skills of experience, understanding, judgment and decision in ethical discourse. Furthermore, the cognitional structure analysis of Lonergan, on its own, does not yield immediate solutions to value conflicts. Cognitional theory provides insights into the four levels of operations. It remains for women and men to draw upon the fruits of the contextualist and proceduralist analyses, as well as upon an appropriation of the four levels of consciousness in concrete instances of ethical deliberation.

The conclusion we draw from this study is that the understanding and responsible management of ethical discourse need to draw upon all three lines of theoretical analysis. Guidelines for moving through the four levels of ethical meaning in the deliberations can be drawn from Lonergan's cognitional theory. Criteria for analyzing the way that social contexts are implicated in cases can be drawn from contextualist analysis. Part 1 of this project, which analyzes the implicit ethics of professionals in health care teams, provides a significant contribution to this work. Finally, criteria for understanding and managing the structural dynamics of the discourse itself can be drawn from proceduralist analysis. The following chapter surveys research results in the field of conflict resolution and offers an important contribution to this line of analysis.

Chapter 8

Value Conflicts in Health Care Teams

Peter Monette

Conflicts among professionals in health care teams often involve differences over values. As was observed in part 1, these value differences are often implicit and are often related to the diverse ways in which professionals of different types understand themselves and their work. The field of conflict resolution has developed a range of insights into the dynamics of conflicts and a range of tools for helping disputants move toward resolution in situations of conflict. In this chapter we will examine some contributions from this field, particularly those contributions that lend themselves to better understanding value conflicts in health care contexts.

The strategy of this chapter will be to begin with a brief introduction to four recognized approaches to conflict resolution that offer resources for understanding and guiding ethical discourse in multiprofessional health care teams. We will proceed to integrate some of the insights from these approaches into the ethical theory framework of Lonergan. We will then move to an extended discussion of the relevance of these resources for the health care setting. Here we will make some linkages with the insights from the analysis of the implicit ethics of professionals from part 1. However, before proceeding, a brief comment on the discussion of ethics and values in the conflict resolution literature is in order.

VALUES AND VALUE CONFLICTS

The goal of this chapter is to examine resources from the field of conflict resolution that can prove helpful in understanding and guiding ethical conflicts in health care. However, when we look to the field of conflict resolution, there seems to be no clear consensus that disputants can come to any agreement on values. Many researchers and practitioners treat values as those sorts of things that are so personal, so intimate and so subjective that no mediation process can offer grounds for agreement. Christopher Moore provides an example. In his analysis, conflicts of interest can generate value disputes that

> focus on such issues as guilt and innocence, what norms should prevail in a social relationship, what facts should be considered valid, what beliefs are correct, who merits what, or what principles should guide decision makers.[1]

For Moore, value conflicts are difficult to resolve because they involve intangibles. It is difficult to negotiate about guilt or social norms. Like Moore, many authors in the field tend to shy away from dealing with values in conflict.

Many theorists and practitioners in the field view values as "the composite record of our life experience and are therefore slow to change."[2] They are private convictions about how to live in our world. Since values are an individual's beliefs about the way the world exists, or should exist, values are non-negotiable. This understanding is rooted in the claims of liberal philosophy that see the individual as the sole determiner of what is valuable. No one can tell someone else what he or she should hold as worthwhile, since one individual's values are equal to those of another. There is no room within conflict resolution to dispute individual values,[3] since conflict resolution is not about changing another person's values or worldviews. The aim of conflict resolution, then, is not to resolve individual value differences. The goal of conflict resolution is to facilitate the cooperative arrangement among disputants in spite of their individual value differences.

Moore is aware that value differences do emerge during the conflict resolution process. For Moore, these value differences emerge because one person attempts to impose his or her value system upon the other person. This occurs because values tend to be associated with intractable feelings and emotions. The intensity of these emotions, when linked with one's values, escalates the conflict to the point that one imposes one's values upon the other. This escalation of the conflict can produce a dispute with extremely locked positions. Within these locked positions each disputant puts forth his or her own way of viewing the world in such a

---

1. Christopher W. Moore, *The Mediation Process: Practical Strategies for Resolving Conflict* (San Francisco: Jossey-Bass, 1986), 174.

2. Susan L. Carpenter and W. J. D. Kennedy, *Managing Public Disputes: A Practical Guide to Handling Conflict and Reaching Agreements* (San Francisco: Jossey-Bass, 1988), 197-198.

3. Fred E. Jandt and P. Gillette, *Win-Win Negotiation: Turning Conflict into Agreement* (New York: John Wiley and Sons, 1985).

way that all alternatives are rejected. This kind of escalated value conflict of opposing worldviews becomes nearly impossible to resolve.

Such views are common in the literature in the field. We would argue, however, that these views represent an overly restrictive understanding of value and an overly narrow view of the way that values function in discourse. What is clear from part 1 is that values take a wide range of forms and often exert their influence implicitly in the discourse process. Often values are about the way professionals view the goals of their practice, the field of concerns that define their practice or the sorts of responsibilities they have toward their patients or clients. Following Lonergan's analysis of the four levels of value, ethical language functions on a variety of levels, ranging from the level of individual desire, through the levels of social and historical order, to the level of practical action strategies. Many of these types of values are regularly disputed in personal and professional contexts and ethical deliberation often finds disputants moving toward agreement on issues rooted in values of various types. Finally, when we open up the meaning of the term "value," we see that many authors in the field of conflict resolution do recognize and promote strategies for moving toward agreement on issues involving values.

We would argue that one of the reasons for this resistance to seeing value conflicts as open to resolution is a view of value that restricts the meaning of the term "value" to those deepest forms of fundamental self-constituting values. To be sure, such values exist and when they come into play they are often quite resistant to change. However, the total range of values is not restricted to fundamental values. And the analyses of the chapters of this volume are offered to help identify when and how values arise in disputes among professionals and how their understanding can help promote effective deliberation toward the resolution of conflicts. In addition, these discussions can help disputants and professionals understand how values are open to argument and analysis. Values have a grounding in experience and are open to reflection and judgment. They are not merely private affairs and the deliberation process is the forum where conflicting values are subjected to analysis in a discourse involving all parties of the team. Finally, even when conflicts in fundamental self-constituting values come into play in a dispute, this need not spell the end of the discourse. As we shall see, conflict analysts and practitioners have developed strategies for transforming relationships among disputants that involve the recognition and respect of differences. Such transformations can provide a foundation for moving beyond blockages and developing action strategies that can prove agreeable to all parties.

AN INTRODUCTION TO SELECTED RESOURCES FROM THE FIELD OF CONFLICT RESOLUTION

Authors often divide approaches to conflict resolution into two groups: position-based approaches and interest-based approaches. Position-based approaches are characterized by an emphasis on settlement, results and outcomes. Disputants come into disputes with conflicting positions and during the dispute they make trade-offs from a hierarchy of positions until they achieve agreement on what they explicitly want. Interest-based, or integrative, approaches, on the other hand, emphasize deeper-level convictions, desires and concerns that often are not easily articulated by the participants themselves. These approaches see disputes over positions as driven by the deeper, more hidden interests and, consequently, see the conflict resolution process as seeking the explicit articulation and mutual recognition of interests.

Christopher Moore's book *The Mediation Process* offers an analysis of the two approaches and proposes an example of the integrative approach. In his discussion of the conflict resolution process, Moore makes the distinction between interests and positions. Positions are the presenting problems that the disputants hold out as the reasons for the conflict. Interests are the underlying needs, wants, desires and values of the disputants. Positions are usually concrete and narrowly defined. Interests are often broad-based and less tangible. This distinction can be used to categorize two kinds of conflicts: conflicts over positions and conflicts over interests. Moore observes that, in his experience, conflicts over positions usually involve underlying interests that are held in common by the disputants. And this commonality can often provide a basis for working out agreement on positions. Even when there are conflicts over interests, there often remain other interests held in common and so the process of probing and explicitly articulating these common interests can provide a platform for moving toward agreement on positions.

Moore uses this insight to argue for an approach to conflict resolution that focusses on the underlying interests. The goal of the resolution process is to probe for these commonly held interests and to articulate them as a basis for an agreement on the positions. The role of the third-party mediator is to help disputants bring these implicitly held interests out into the open, and to mutually recognize them. The result of this mutual recognition is an opening up of the process of discourse in the dispute to a state where the parties can look for mutually agreeable solutions to the issues involved in the positions.

Fisher and Keashly offer a similar analysis of the field.[4] Their analysis of the literature on third-party interventions in conflicts distinguishes between mediation and problem solving. The basic difference between problem solving (also called conciliation) and mediation exists in their different underlying assumptions about conflict. Mediation tends to view conflict as a matter of differing goals or values (objective differences). Problem solving or conciliation tends to view conflict as a misperception and misunderstanding between parties (subjective differences). Although any conflict may include both these dimensions, the processes of mediation and conciliation will focus predominantly on one or another of these dimensions.

The authors argue that the traditional mediation approach will "accept a competitive, win–lose orientation and concentrate on developing a compromise."[5] The focus is on the objective dimension of the conflict while working around relationship issues. Problem-solving conflict resolution, however, will focus on the basic relationship of the disputants. It assumes "that reevaluation of perceptions, attitudes, behaviours and priorities will facilitate a more collaborative and integrative approach to the resolution of the more objective issues."[6] Thus, where a mediator will use reasoning, persuasion and control of both process and substantive issues, the problem solver or conciliator will use process-orientated human skills to guide her intervention. Fisher and Keashly write that

> The essence of third party consultations involves the interventions of a skilled and impartial intermediary who attempts to facilitate creative problem solving by improving communications and analysing the underlying issues and the relationship between the parties.[7]

This move to the relationship in effect alters the understanding of the conflict for each disputant. From this new understanding of their conflict, disputants are able to address the objective dimension of their conflict.

While differences exist between Moore's approach and that of Fisher and Keashly, what is of interest is their similar focus on probing beyond immediate presenting problems toward deeper, implicitly held convictions that can provide a basis for renewing relationships and rebuilding discourse. These authors present insights and strategies for transforming

---

4. Ron J. Fisher and L. Keashly, "Third Party Interventions in Intergroup Conflict: Consultation is *Not* Mediation," *Negotiation Journal* 4, no. 4 (1988): 381-393.

5. Ibid., 382.

6. Ibid., 381.

7. Ibid., 382.

conflicts into discourse that can move the parties toward common understanding and action.

Another approach that focusses on the transformation of disputes has been put forward by Dukes.[8] Early in 1993 Dukes wrote his reflections on the state of public conflict resolution after his experience at the 1992 conference of the Society of Professionals in Dispute Resolution (SPIDR). Dukes maintains that the current practice of conflict resolution is in crisis. The crisis can be summarized as a conflict over two different visions of public conflict resolution. The first, or "traditional," vision, Dukes calls "management ideology." The second, Dukes' preferred model, is called "transformative public conflict resolution."

Dukes argues that the current trend in public conflict resolution operates with a management vision. The management vision proposes public conflict resolution in order to save money, reduce court costs, eliminate delays and reduce the demands on government. Dukes argues that the management vision parallels the political emphasis on utilitarianism.[9] Public conflict resolution becomes a means of distributing political power among the various special interest groups, the select players in the conflict resolution process. This being so, the management vision limits the range of available problems to be discussed and solutions to be found to those within the domain of the existing participants. And the management vision effectively limits the discourse to those "at the table."

For Dukes, the transformative model of public conflict resolution has a much wider vision. It sees the role of public conflict resolution as "not limited to the settlement of disputes; rather, it is a vehicle for changing governing practices and the institutional culture of agencies, public officials, citizenry and communities."[10]

Transformative public conflict resolution attempts to create an engaged community involved in a public discourse "that empowers people to articulate their needs freely and to explore their differences fairly."[11] It attempts to achieve a civic consciousness where individuals "are capable of transcending limitations of self-interest in search for common goals."[12]

---

8.   Frank Dukes, "Public Conflict Resolution: A Transformative Approach," *Negotiation Journal* 9, no. 1 (1993): 45-57.

9.   Dukes refers to Jürgen Habermas as a writer who addresses similar concerns about contemporary society. For Habermas' discourse ethics, see his *Moral Consciousness and Communicative Action*, trans. C. Lenhardt and S. Nicholsen (Cambridge: MIT Press, 1991).

10. Dukes, "Public Conflict Resolution," 47.

11. Ibid., 47-48.

12. Ibid., 49.

This can be achieved by focussing on relationships with bonds of acceptance and responsibility.

Dukes' model understands disputes as "socially constituted, dynamic mechanisms, whose actors, issues and consequences are invariably shaped and transformed by the means available, offered and used to contest them."[13] Thus, it focusses on sustaining the relationships among the disputants. It looks toward a transformation in public policy from an attitude of self-interest to one of common welfare. The relatedness dimension triggers a host of other elements, such as responsibility, obligation, loyalty, respect, recognition, mutuality, understanding and empathy.

A fourth set of authors addressing the issue of transformation in conflict resolution is Bush and Folger. Their ground-breaking book *The Promise of Mediation: Responding to Conflict Through Empowerment and Recognition*[14] offers an alternative understanding to the practice of mediation. The authors argue that mediation is currently being practised through a settlement model that focusses upon problem solving at the expense of the relationship among the disputants. For Bush and Folger the process of mediation offers more than simply a way for people to problem solve their conflicts. Mediation can be viewed as a process within which disputants can be morally transformed. Bush and Folger offer the Transformative Model as a place for mutual discovery and moral growth. Their argument rests upon an understanding of moral development as represented by two dimensions: justice and care. The authors attempt an integration of these basic orientations of moral development, which they call "compassionate strength." Compassionate strength is an integration of concerns for self and concerns for the other. In mediation this means that the disputants can change in ways that reflect both dimensions of moral growth. Appropriate moral attention of the disputants and the mediator must focus on both one's own concerns and one's concerns for the other disputant. Bush and Folger argue that such focus can be promoted in mediation by attention to two corresponding dimensions: empowerment and recognition. Empowerment means strengthening one's self-determination and self-reliance. Recognition means relating to the other through respect and consideration of the other's needs. The goal of mediation under the Transformative Model is to foster "secure and self-reliant beings willing to be concerned with and responsive to others (strong and caring)."[15] This approach to mediation anticipates the possibility of

---

13. Ibid., 50.

14. Robert Baruch Bush and Joseph Folger, *The Promise of Mediation: Responding to Conflict Through Empowerment and Recognition* (San Francisco: Jossey-Bass, 1994).

15. Bush and Folger, *The Promise of Mediation*, 29

moral change within the disputants through the process of resolving their differences.

The common theme running through the authors examined here is a vision of conflict resolution as a structured process where disputants can move from the explicit issues that are creating conflict and blocking discourse to a focus on deeper, underlying issues that can provide a common ground for constructive discourse. In one way or another, the authors recognize a distinction between explicit issues and implicit issues and they see the move to the articulation of implicit issues as the route through conflicts, toward common understanding and action. This line of analysis supports the overall approach of this study and promises resources for helping teams of health care professionals in their ethical deliberations. Moreover, it offers support for the strategy of clarifying the implicit values operative in the self-understanding of health care professionals and suggests ways that these clarifications could prove helpful in the ethical deliberation process.

The next step in this analysis, then, is to understand the link between the general orientation of conflict resolution and the particular insights into the structure of ethics in the work of Bernard Lonergan. Once this is clarified, the ethical framework can help understand how the more precise insights from conflict resolution can shed light on the interactions among health care professionals.

BERNARD LONERGAN'S NOTION OF VALUE AND THE STRUCTURE OF VALUE CONFLICTS

Bernard Lonergan offers us a comprehensive conceptualization of the nature and function of value.[16] We can schematize Lonergan's approach by considering value as functioning on four levels. The first is the level of individual needs and desires. Individuals are originators of values and these values are initially experienced prethematically as feelings. One's feelings express convictions about ourselves and our world. These felt values structure the ways in which an individual perceives the world. This is the common-sense understanding of values, because this is what is usually understood and acted on.

This order of value as feelings expressing needs and desires can lead to a further level of value. Feelings are intentional responses to values in human situations. This is to say that feelings intend the creation of some

---

16. See Chapter 6 by Kenneth R. Melchin for more details.

good. Now, this good is particular as far as it concerns concrete goods.[17] But this second level of value rests upon the insight that the host of individual needs and desires cannot be met by an individual alone. This insight objectifies the prethematic feelings as goods to be realized. In other words, the fulfilment of individual needs and desires requires the help of other individuals. When individuals come together to help each other fulfil their own individual needs and desires, they do so through cooperation. The cooperative structure among individuals is the setup within which individuals may become satisfied in their needs and desires.

This cooperative structure or setup is what Lonergan has named "the good of order" and it is the second level of value.[18] The good of order is meant to achieve that which has been expressed by the feelings of participating individuals. The living arrangement of the cooperative structure allows for the possibility that the participating individuals will establish a set of shared meaning.[19] This common set of meaning includes the sharing of anticipations and expectations among each other during their cooperative enterprises. This common set of meaning becomes a necessary

---

17. The point is that the good of order is not simply some utilitarian concept meant to produce an aggregate of material goods for a given group of people. The good of order contributes to the humanizing character of human living by creating and ordering nonmaterial values such as trust, openness and mutuality.

18. There are four general characteristics of the good of order. First, the good of order is meant to provide for the satisfaction of needs and desires not just once, but continuously. The good of order is a setup for the regular recurrence of some good. Second, the good of order arranges the organization of human operations. Individuals participate within the good of order according to a specific arrangement with the aim of creating a particular good. Third, the good of order is conditioned by habits, institutions and material. Habits are cognitional and volitional. Participants in the good of order must already know, must already be willing and must have the appropriate skills for the proper functioning of the good of order. Institutions must be in place for the facilitation of the delivery of the particular good. Institutions contribute to the socialization of individuals whereby members of a society may cooperate on a social level without a movement to a personal level. The good of order requires material equipment. The good of order needs buildings, vehicles, computers, paper and pens. The fourth general characteristic is personal status. The good of order configures the roles of the cooperating individuals. People take on roles within relationships according to the nature of the social recurrence scheme. Associated with these roles are sets of expectations manifested in the relationship by the sequence of gestures and responses. Through this sequence participants are able to create shared meaning by the reciprocal role taking place in the cooperation. But this recurrence is neither a matter of randomness, nor mechanical configuration. The regular recurrence of a particular good of order is configured by a set of exigencies. This set includes, for example, the integrity of the participants, cultural and religious values and field-specific conditions. The good of order functions according to a factor of probability that it will generate the appropriate good. See Bernard Lonergan, *Topics in Education* (Toronto: University of Toronto Press, 1993), 33-37; *Insight*, 596; and *Method in Theology*, 47-51.

condition for the possibility that the participants will cooperate in the creation of their good of order.

The third level of value involves a judgment of both the worthwhileness of the good of order and the goods that flow from the cooperative structure. This judgment involves judging the good of order from a wider historical perspective. The good of order is judged as truly valuable when it contributes to the humanization of the social order viewed from within a wider historical perspective. And this goal of articulating the commonly held aspirations about the social good is what is sought in the process of ethical deliberation.

The fourth level refers to the set of actions and responsibilities that emerges from this wider vision of social, historical value. This level of value attempts to realize the commonly held values that are affirmed in the collective judgment of values of the participants. Taken together, the four levels of value attempt to express the complex nature of how value is affirmed in ethical discourse.

To borrow an example from Lonergan, we all have a need to eat breakfast. We need to eat breakfast not only this morning, but every morning. The social setup to bring breakfast to everyone's table is the good of order. This good of order organizes participants into social relationships; there are farmers and merchants, bakers and butchers. Each has a role to play according to one's specific habits and skills.[20] Each is organized into institutions, like marketing boards, meant to facilitate the flow of goods. We are all, then, able to eat breakfast not just once but every morning. And so, the recurrent experience of breakfast each morning is judged as a good event because it is a condition for the emergence of both particular goods and authentic human beings.

However, not all setups are truly good. Some are oppressive, others exclude minorities, others create havoc for future generations. Consequently the deliberation process must move to the third level to scrutinize social orders and find and correct their flaws. Finally, this evaluative process must issue in action strategies that respond to the problems at hand. And so the deliberation process must move to the fourth level of value, informed by some common vision of the overall project that sets the context for the contributions of all participants.

---

19. For a more analytical discussion of the sharing of meaning, see Kenneth R. Melchin, "Moral Knowledge and the Structure of Cooperative Living," *Theological Studies* 52 (1991): 495-523, especially his discussion on the basic social scheme of human discourse, where he borrows from the work of Gibson Winter and George Hubert Mead.

20. This arrangement of roles involves the authentic meaning made by each participant. This meaning is constitutive of the way each person actually lives one's role within the good of order.

We can use Lonergan's understanding of value to more fully grasp how insights from the field of conflict resolution can contribute to the understanding of ethical deliberation. Through this analysis we hope to move beyond a limited understanding of value that views value as solely individual feelings toward the fourfold level of value presented above. The following section will describe methods of resolving conflicts of value that have been suggested by practitioners in the field of conflict resolution. We will build on this by drawing on insights into the transformation occurring in conflict resolution and the stages in the mediation process and integrating these within the framework provided by Lonergan.

When conflicts involve a degree of value differences, Moore suggests three techniques for resolution. First, dissensus issues can be reframed.[21] The reframing of dissensus issues involves the discovery of common interests. For Moore, this is often possible because conflicts are rarely only about values and because interests can usually accommodate a wide range of positions. The skill in this kind of reframing is the ability to move the conflict to the level of the disputants' needs and desires. It is often the case that what appears to be opposing positions at the presenting level are common interests at the level of needs and desires. This is generally described in the mediation literature as achieving common ground. It is the process of going deeper to the underlying or foundational aspects of the disputants. An integrative conflict resolution process fosters the recognition by all parties that they do share more in common than their conflict. Going deeper is one way of dealing with value differences. Going higher is another way. Going higher is Moore's second technique, which he calls a search for superordinate values. This search aims to achieve a mutual recognition by the disputants that there are more important values to be created through their cooperative participation. This search is facilitated by designing a hierarchy of values agreeable by all the disputants. With the higher values in sight, the lower values can then be translated. This translation becomes the core of the mediation session as the disputants work out a settlement. The third technique is simply the agreement among the disputants to "agree to disagree." For Moore, it is not necessary that every conflict of value be resolved before disputants live in a cooperative arrangement. Most often, in fact, we live with others with quite different understandings of the way the world should be. We therefore agree that we disagree about some values in order that we can get on with the business of living out of other values. Thus, Moore suggests that conflicts over values can either: (1) be translated into common

---

21. Moore, *The Mediation Process*, 172-186. This chapter relies heavily on the article by V. Aubert, "Competition and Dissensus: Two Types of Conflict and Conflict Resolution," *Journal of Conflict Resolution* 7, no. 1 (1963): 26-42.

interests; (2) become searches for higher common values; or (3) become moments when disputants agree to disagree about their conflicting values in order to resolve their practical differences.

I would suggest that these three techniques result in the same end but in different ways. The first two of these three techniques to resolving difference of value is a difference in conceptualization. A movement to basic common interests as expressed as common needs, desires and values is the same as a search for superordinate values as common values linking subordinate values. The first technique looks downward to fundamental, underlying or common ground among the disputants. The second technique looks upward to common values that may inspire and bond other lower conflicting values among the disputants. The third technique of avoiding the difference of value or "agreeing to disagree" about a conflict over values is achieved only by the recognition among the disputants that they have a common interest or a superordinate value to their conflicting value, that is, the value or need of getting on with the business of living.

What becomes clear is that Moore's approach aims at restoring and sustaining the cooperative arrangement among the disputants. I would argue that he tends to avoid dealing with the values that are conflictual because these values cannot be dealt with in the short term. When values are understood as being about an individual's worldview, beliefs and normative expectations, one can understand how one would not want to deal with them when one's basic goal is to arrive at a cooperative settlement for the short term.

However, there are many relationships that are long-term. Often workplace relationships are sustained over months, years, even decades. Recurrent interrelationships involved in human living necessitate the movement toward more creative attempts at both understanding and resolving value differences.[22] In order to work this out, however, we will need to operate from a more comprehensive understanding of the nature and function of value.

---

22. Part of this argument rests upon the concern that conflict resolution process, like mediation, does not resolve the structural arrangement among disputants. Lack of attention to the structural level generates chronic conflict and multiple use of the mediation process. Perhaps part of this lack of attention to the structural arrangement of the disputants is due to the mediator's narrow understanding of value. Understanding values to include the structural arrangement of the disputants could help in resolving chronic conflict based upon structural problematics. See for example, H. Mika, "Social Conflict, Local Justice: Organizational Responses to the Astructural Bias," *Supplement to Interaction*, Publication of the Network Interaction for Conflict Resolution 4 (Spring 1992): 1-4.

Our concern with continual or sustained relationships and our need for a comprehensive understanding of value allows us to integrate Lonergan's notion of value with the transformation that can occur during a dispute-resolution process. Lonergan's fourfold notion of value allows us to understand that value is more than the individual belief system of the disputant. The disputants' interaction or structural arrangement involves the good of order within which they manifest their humanity and with which they may become satisfied in their needs and interests. The conflictual nature of their relationship means that their good of order is not functioning in line with their needs. The process of conflict resolution is the facilitation of the disputants' creative response to their dysfunctional arrangement. The process of conflict resolution, depending as it does upon the structure of communication, consists of a wide range of values that are held by all disputants.[23] From this agreed set of values the disputants work with a third party to correct their particular setup. The process of this correction requires that disputants move through a transformative shift consisting in a new understanding that their own needs and interests cannot be met without their cooperative arrangement. This is expressed as the shift from "I want" statements to "we want" statements. This shift is "within" the individual as much as it is a new perspective founded upon a common set of shared meaning. This shift is "without" the individual as much as it is the condition of possibility that the disputants will be able to create a new and better cooperative setup. The disputants must reach a judgment about this new cooperative setup. This settlement includes identifying any new relationships and sets of responsibility that are deemed necessary in order to carry out the settlement. The judgment of the new arrangement occurs both during the conflict resolution process and continuously during the actual operation of the settlement. During the lived experience of their new arrangement the disputants will continue to make judgments about the worthwhileness of their arrangement. When the worthwhileness of their cooperative arrangement is put into doubt, a new conflict will begin to emerge and the process of conflict and conflict resolution will begin once again.

Our understanding of the four levels of value can be discerned within the structure of the mediation process.[24] Typically, mediation consists of

---

23. Conflicts involve both procedural and substantive elements. See chapter 6 by James Sauer in this book.

24. For the purposes of this illustration, we will assume that the conflict involves two disputants and one mediator. The basic stages presented would be used in more complex conflicts.

four stages.[25] The *introduction stage* sets up the interaction among the disputants and the mediator. This stage consists in an agreement among the parties regarding both the process to be followed and the ground rules to be applied. This stage establishes a set of shared procedural values recognized by each disputant. For example, the procedure of mediation illustrates the common value judgment that discourse is a better way of resolving their dispute than violence. The *second stage* of mediation consists in identifying the positions and interests of the disputants. From a transformative perspective this stage is the heart of mediation. During this stage the mediator will focus on the process of the discourse. The mediator will, for example, intervene when the rules of discourse, mutually agreed upon in stage one, have been broken by one or both disputants. The aim of this stage is to achieve the movement from positions to interests. In other words, the disputants begin the mediation session with their presenting problem. This is usually expressed as their reason for conflict. It is generically expressed as an "I want" statement. Each disputant typically will have an opening position that expresses his or her individual wants. At this point in the mediation session the disputants are usually set in opposition to one another. There is a perceived disparity between the disputants. The mediation process aims at moving the disputants beyond this rather narrow position. The movement is toward the commonality between the disputants. Each disputant has a wide range of interests supporting their individual position. This wide range of interests allows for a creative search for commonality or common ground. The creative commonality is the foundation for the new arrangement that will emerge between the disputants. This becomes expressed as a "we want" statement. This statement reflects the recognition between the disputants that their interests can only be met by their cooperative arrangement. This cooperative arrangement, impossible before mediation, is now possible because the disputants recognize and acknowledge each other's needs and interests. Such recognition and acknowledgment is the necessary condition for the establishment of their new arrangement.

The movement from positions to underlying interests can be facilitated by the mediator through her repertoire of skills. This dialogical movement attempts to allow the disputants to shift from their narrow "I want" positions to their common "we want" interests. The mediator will facilitate this shift by controlling the discourse. The mediator's language

---

25. The four stages I have identified are adapted from C. A. Picard, *Campus Mediation Training Manual* (Ottawa: Carleton University Press, 1993). Picard divides mediation into five stages: (1) Introduce the process; (2) Identify the issues; (3) Explore the issues; (4) Generate solutions; (5) Reach agreement. Stages 2 and 3 are separated in the actual mediation session in order to control the discourse. They are, in fact, part of the same stage that I have identified as the movement from positions to interests.

skills include such techniques as reframing, restating and probing. The *third stage* of mediation is the search for a precise description of the disputants' intention for a new creative arrangement. Typically called "brainstorming," the disputants seek out ways that their common and individual needs and interests can be met in equitable means. This stage usually brings about arrangements that were unimaginable before the mediation session because of the emotional distance that separated the disputants. The *fourth stage* is the actual settlement. From the many possible solutions, the disputants must choose the best arrangement. This stage involves a common substantive judgment that a particular arrangement will in fact meet the needs and interests of both parties. Mediation has satisfied their needs of discourse (versus the possible alternative of violence) and the settlement meets their needs of cooperation necessary to fulfil their originating needs that were once in conflict. The stage is finalized in a written contract. This contract sets up the range of expectations that each disputant can anticipate from each other in terms of mutual relationships and responsibility. Mediation, therefore, represents a dialogical moment in the relationship of the disputants—a moment that reconfigures not only their structural arrangement but also their recognition of each other as interrelated individuals who require mutual cooperation for their continual living.

APPLICATION TO THE HEALTH CARE SETTING

The basic structure of discourse organized in the stages of mediation shows that there is a value transformation occurring during the resolution of conflict. The value transformation involves the creation of a shared meaning framework that shifts the disputants' original conflict position from an individually oriented perspective toward a common viewpoint. The following is presented as a brief description of a value transformation that can occur during an ethical conflict between a doctor and a nurse. In this discussion we will begin to integrate some of the insights from part 1 on the implicit ethics of health care professionals. What becomes clear from this illustration is how the implicit ethics associated with diverse professionals' conceptions of their roles and tasks function to skew the deliberation process, and how our analytic tools can help to get the deliberation process on track.

Imagine that a nurse and a doctor are in a conflict over the procedure of a particular treatment for a certain patient. Both professionals know that the treatment will be painful. But they disagree over the possible success of this treatment. The nurse and the doctor view the conflict from different perspectives or horizons,[26] perspectives that are rooted in their own implicit professional ethos. This horizon or perspective tends to delimit their range of possible knowledge and interests. Both professionals claim the same first-level value to be in the best interest of the patient.

Let us say that the doctor's implicit professional ethos is defined by the traditional "Expert" type, the first of the models analyzed in part 1, the model that views the physician as sole decision maker. And let us say that the nurse's horizon is defined by a combination of types. In part she reflects the "Advocate" type, which views nurses more traditionally as subservient to the doctor in terms of treatment decision making. But this kind of role relationship is quickly changing. The nurse's horizon is taking on elements of the "Manager" type, which claims a role in decision making. There is the beginning of a view that she might be more equal to the physician. This greater sense of equality is freeing her to function more autonomously as the patient's "Advocate."[27] Associated with the ethos or horizon of each is a range of interests, feelings and emotions.

Now, each professional addresses the problem as if their own horizon were the proper or true horizon. This results in a clash of values between these professionals. Each one sees only a part or subset of the total range of values involved in the larger situation. Conflict between the professionals escalates when their emotions rise as each professional attempts to defend their respective horizon. Such defence produces entrenched, intractable positions and chronic conflict patterns over time. Yet the nurse's and the doctor's horizons can, in fact, be complementary to each other. Discovering the grounds for this complementarity is essential for the movement to the second level of values and the development of common action strategies.

The professional relationship between the nurse and the doctor demands that they work together. Their professional relationship structures how they will interact. But this structure is dependent upon the doctor and the nurse. Together they must create this structure within the limits of the larger hospital institutional structure, yet they have each approached

---

26. The introduction of the concept of "horizon" in necessitated by the professionalization of the disputants (nursing and medicine). This requires a greater control of the perspectives held by each disputant. Lonergan describes a horizon as the limits of one's field of vision. Within one's horizon lies one's interests and one's knowledge. Lying beyond one's horizon one neither knows nor cares. Horizons condition one's standpoint, knowledge and interests. They are in turn conditioned by the historical period one lives within, by one's social background, one's education and one's personal development. See chapter 10, "Dialectics," *Method in Theology*, 235 ff.

27. See H. J. Schattschneider, "Power Relationships Between Physician and Nurse," *Humane Medicine* 6, no. 3 (1990): 197-201.

the problem from within their particular professional horizons. The shift to the second order of value is dependent upon the twofold insight that their horizons are complementary and that they cannot achieve their common goal without their collaborative arrangement.[28] Neither the doctor nor the nurse *can individually* achieve the overall best interest of the patient. This insight of collaboration requires the creation of a set of shared meaning between these two professionals.

This mutual set of meanings will represent an integration of their previously clashing horizons.[29] This integration is facilitated by a movement toward a higher viewpoint: the perspective of the patient within a consideration of the wider institutional health care setting. It is this wider perspective that can orientate, or integrate, the professionals' horizons such that there emerges a common, shared set of meanings.[30] Probing the full implications of this emergence can involve a real transformation for the professionals. Each must move from their original horizons to the new common horizon integrated by the wider vision of the patient's perspective. This common horizon is a condition of possibility that the professionals will be able to work out a collaborative structure for their professional interactions.

This new good of order among the professionals is a different form of professional ethos. It recognizes the respective value contributions that come from the practices and commitments of the other professionals involved in care. And it arises to the extent that the implicit values of the diverse professions are raised to explicit consciousness and acknowledged. It sets the stage for new working relationships and sets of corresponding responsibilities. Working out this new set of professional values can be done through the process of integrative conflict resolution. Conflict resolution offers some techniques, such as reframing, that

---

28. To be effective over the long term, the resolution of this ethical conflict must address the structural arrangement between professionals throughout the hospital. In this way, the mechanisms of conflict resolution will be attentive to both the individual level of the particular disputants and the larger institutional level involving every doctor and nurse.

29. This integration has been identified by Pike as a kind of synergy among the health care professionals. Adele W. Pike, "Moral Outrage and Moral Discourse in Nurse–Physician Collaboration," *Journal of Professional Nursing* 7, no. 6 (November 1991): 351-363.

30. This is not to be misunderstood as a more complex argument for patients' rights. Patients' rights arguments can tend to be just as fragmented as any other narrowly defined perspective. Rather, the value transformation that can occur during discourse involves *all participants* as each moves through the discourse scheme in attention to their desires and interests, intelligently discerning their new goods of order and making the judgment of the worthwhileness of their cooperative living.

can facilitate the creation of both the shared meaning and the new co-operative arrangement.

Obviously this example is simplified. Real-life conflicts among professionals can be more complicated. The number of interrelationships, for example, multiply to include a discourse among the patient, his or her family and a range of other health care professionals. It is precisely these complexities of real life that demand that we pay closer attention to the dynamics at play. Long-term relationships necessitate attention to conflicting values. They require that disputants reexamine their cooperative setup that aims at creating these values. No doubt this is a time-consuming process. It requires a great deal of communication and repeated attempts at good will. Its fruit is the establishment of a transformation of the participants in their collaborative efforts at creating new meanings and new ways of interacting. And these new ways are meant for the re-current satisfaction of their individual and mutual goals.

We have been discussing the nature and function of value in the resolution of conflicts. We have seen that value is a dynamic concept that incorporates four levels. These levels of value allow us to see that the resolution of conflict requires each of the disputants come to specific values that are shared among them. These shared values become the condition of possibility that the disputants will be able to live their lives in a cooperative way. This set of shared values emerging from the resolution process is *a priori* as far as it develops from the common ground that exists among the disputants. It is *a posteriori* as far as it is something new that is created by the disputants that could not have been thought of before the resolution process. The new set of shared values as both individual and shared and as manifest in their new cooperative arrangement becomes the contours of their actual lived experience. Where once the disputants were conflictual, now they are cooperative; where once they were adversarial, now they are partners in a new and better living arrangement. And this transformation involves raising the implicit values operative in the ethos of professionals to a level of explicit awareness and analysis in the context of ethical deliberation.

There are, however, a number of questions remaining. How can the structure of discourse used to resolve ethical conflicts with particular disputants be used to address larger institutional problematics? What about the issue of consensual notions of truth that were not addressed in this essay?[31] How can power imbalances, embedded as they are in professional roles, be overcome during the resolution process when there is no third party to facilitate the dispute? What exactly is the new integrative perspective generated by the patient's point of view? Are there not at least

---

31. For a discussion of this question, see chapter 6 by James Sauer.

some values that are always conflictual and beyond integration? To answer some of these questions we will turn to a range of insights from the study of conflicts in the health care setting.

REVIEW OF RESEARCH ON CONFLICT RESOLUTION IN HEALTH CARE

The systemic employment of conflict management or facilitation techniques in the health care setting is a recent practice. This practice has emerged in part because of the increasing use of conflict management processes in the workplace and because of the changing roles of health care professionals. The change in roles amounts to a more collaborative model of professional interaction. Such collaboration inevitably involves dealing with different kinds of professional "types" and the conflicts that result from the interactions among these "types." This, in turn, requires the use of the best conflict management techniques currently available. This section will survey some recent attempts at integrating conflict management techniques and processes into the health care setting. First, we will look at suggestions that some professional health care roles are more suited to the task of conflict resolution than others. Second, we will investigate how hospital ethics committees have begun to use various conflict management processes in function of their mandate. Finally, we will survey how the collaborative model of health care professional interaction employs conflict management skills and processes to resolve conflicts about treatment, team interaction and ethical dilemmas.

From the analysis of professional roles, some have suggested that nurses and social workers have the specific responsibility of conflict management. Clearly, the analysis of professional "types" from part 1 would seem to suggest that some "types" are more suited to this role than others. Both Broom and Case[32] suggest that the nurse is the health care professional who most often needs to use conflict management skills because of his or her close proximity to the patient. In her article, Broom puts forth the view that nurses in critical care settings have an opportunity and a responsibility to establish an environment where conflicts concerning the nature of health care (i.e., ethical dilemmas) can be effectively managed for strategic action. She begins by describing a case study involving the positions and feelings of various participants: patient,

---

32. C. Broom, "Conflict Resolution Strategies: When Ethical Dilemmas Evolve into Conflict," *Dimensions of Critical Care Nursing* 10, no. 6 (1991): 354-363; and N. K. Case, "Substituted Judgment in the Pediatric Health Care Setting," *Issues in Comprehensive Pediatric Nursing* 11 (1988): 303-312.

family, nurses, physician and community. From this case, Broom describes six sources of conflict. *Values* are beliefs considered to be true. They are either personal or professional. Personal values pertain to the individual's concept of what is right and morally correct. Professional values are principles that have universal application. These are gleaned from a variety of viewpoints, not biased by personal values, across our pluralistic society. *Perception* concerns the amount of knowledge one has of the situation, one's degree of involvement and the stress one feels in the situation. *Motivation* is the desire one has to act. It can be either internal or external. Internal motivations are one's own commitments. They can be, for example, either paternalistic or maternalistic. External motivations concern factors beyond the individual, for example, fears of litigation. *Responsibility for decisions and actions* refers to such questions as "Who decides?" and "What is to be done?" Broom argues that patients have the right and responsibility to make decisions about their health care. Doctors are responsible for the appropriate course of treatment. Traditionally, patients have given their decision-making power over to their doctors. Difficulties arise when the patient's decision-making capacity is distorted, which often leaves family members responsible for the patient. *Competition for resources* involves the problem of limited resources. "Health care providers must be content with limits that impede their ability to achieve all that is desirable."[33] Conflicts emerge about the costs of highly technological interventions versus prevention programs, or between the kind of health care services to be performed and the available resources. *Incompatible goals* refer to the priorities of treatment that arise from the above factors.

Conflict resolution strategies can help in sorting out the difficulties that emerge from these different sources of conflict. Broom offers strategies in four different levels of intervention. She offers these strategies as tips for critical care nurses who think that their settings need conflict resolution for their ethical dilemmas. On the personal level, Broom suggests that the nurse understand his or her own approach to conflict.[34] This is especially important since ethical dilemmas are often simply avoided by nurses, and this may be related to their approach to conflict.[35] Broom recommends that nurses become familiar with four major ethical frameworks: deontologist, utilitarian, right-based and situation ethics. She also suggests to clarify boundaries, personal and professional, and to be open

---

33. Broom, "Conflict Resolution Strategies," 357.

34. For example, Broom outlines Thomas and Kilmann's styles of conflict resolution. There are five general means of resolving interpersonal conflict: competing, compromising, collaborating, avoiding and accommodating.

35. Broom, "Conflict Resolution Strategies," 359, 361.

to other points of view. On the health care team level, Broom maintains that professionals should share information. They may wish to follow the model of Jonsen, Siegler and Winsdale on the collection and organization of pertinent information.[36] These authors categorize information into four classes: medical condition, patient preference, quality of life and external factors. She also recommends that professionals acknowledge differences to promote the group process. The team needs to identify desired outcomes and objectives in order to avoid personal biases. Finally, she recommends that the team attempt to reach consensus through shared priorities. On the organizational level, Broom recommends that nurses be trained in conflict resolution techniques, that there be a nurses' ethics committee or group and that nurses make use of their psychosocial clinical nurse specialist. On the community level, Broom suggests that the community interest be assessed, that the community be educated and that nurses participate in their community's public policy regarding health care allocation.

Case puts forth the argument that it is the role of the nurse to facilitate between the best interests of the patient and the other members of the health care team. Although she does not say that the nurse should mediate among these professionals, she does describe the nurse's role with adjectives similar to those used to describe mediators. Case writes that in the example of substituted judgment in pediatric patients, the nurse should "assess patients' understanding of the situation, identify information needs and assist parents to articulate their needs and desires to the rest of the health care team."[37] Yet Case is aware of the emotional investment of all those involved in any particular case. In the situation of substituted judgment, there are two extremes to be avoided: autonomy of the patient and autonomy of the physician. Case writes, "a means must be made available for negotiation of disputed positions."[38] Case suggests that no one person, either parent or professional, should be the sole proxy of a child facing life-and-death issues. There is the need, therefore, to set up a means of negotiation among interested parties before the situation reaches the legal stage. As part of the solution, Case makes the claim that this could be achieved through using an ideal ethical observer. This involves a balanced resolution of conflicts between health care professionals and the parents in cases of substituted judgment.[39] The ideal ethical observer consists of four components. First,

---

36. A. Jonsen, M. Siegler and W. Winslade, *Clinical Ethics*, 2nd ed. (New York: Macmillan, 1986).

37. Case, "Substituted Judgment," 305.

38. Ibid., 307.

this person would be *omniscient* in that all pertinent information would be made available. Second, the person would be *omnipercipient* in that the feelings of all involved would be taken into consideration. This in-

---

39. The question of "Who decides?" is a tenacious issue in health care ethics. Case's argument is supported in part by Robert Burt in his book *Taking Care of Strangers* (New York: Free Press, 1979).

Burt argues that the current debate regarding doctor–patient relations sets up a false dichotomy between either the doctor as sole choice maker and the patient as choiceless, or the doctor as choiceless and the patient as autonomous decision maker. Burt argues that this is a false dichotomy, because it does not address the intrapsychic reality of the self/other boundaries. The dichotomy falsely establishes these boundaries as either too rigid or as enmeshed. He says that fixed boundaries "disregard the bonds of mutual recognition that underlie everyone's sense of individuality, of the intrapsychic process by which self and other are depicted" (42).

Establishing these boundaries as enmeshed leads to a choice maker/choiceless arrangement whereby the doctor or judge is the sole decision maker. This false dichotomy has led to *brutality* in the health care profession, because the pain in the other invokes pain for the self. One's response is to remove the source of the pain. Burt elaborates this intrapsychic conflict via Freudian psychoanalysis. Therefore, the intrapsychic boundary between doctor and patient must never be conclusively settled (121). It is this intrapsychic argument that grounds Burt's entire work. He sums it up this way: "Rules governing doctor–patient relations must rest on the premise that anyone's wish to help a desperately pained, apparently helpless person is intertwined with a wish to hurt that person, to obliterate him from sight" (vi).

Current civil commitment laws, for example, rest upon categories such as mental normality, mentally ill, retarded and comatose. But, in making these decisions, law makers must keep in mind that "every individual—whether 'diseased person,' physician, or judge—has difficulty in fixing himself within these categories and how that difficulty creates tensions between benevolent and abusive impulses toward himself and others" (vii).

Burt develops this thesis through the use of various case studies. Mr. G. concerns the issue of patient rights. Mrs. Lake concerns the issue of doctor/state as the decision maker. The infamous Milgram experiments emphasize subject powerlessness to benevolent authority. The final two case studies, Quinlan and Saikewicz, involve the issue of a silent patient.

Burt proposes that the best way to prevent the horrors of this false dichotomy is a greater range of conversation among the parties involved. The proper role of the courts, or third parties, is not as decision maker, but as promoter of rational discourse among the participants (121). There must be no sole decision maker (20-21). The decision-making space is the framework of the conversation among all those involved (122). This conversation may be very time-consuming, difficult, uncomfortable and even painful for those involved. Yet it is the best way to be sure that the good intentions of the health care professions, legal professions and patients' rights advocates do not become hurtful and horrifying responses.

For a discussion of "Who decides?," or third-order decision making, see F. Schauer, "The Right to Die as a Case Study in Third-Order Decision Making," *The Journal of Medicine and Philosophy* 17 (1992): 573-587.

cludes the range of psychosocial factors like cultural and religious values. Third, the ideal ethical observer would be *disinterested*. This person would not have a vested interest in the dispute. Fourth, the person would be *dispassionate* or, at least, less emotionally involved in the dispute. Although Case does not write how the ideal ethical observer would proceed, she does maintain that the ideal ethical observer would not have a decision-making capacity. Case suggests that since no one person could possibly have these characteristics, the ideal ethical observer would actually be a group of professionals. Case, however, is not clear about how this might be worked out. She ends her article by claiming that nurses are possibly the professionals best suited for this role, since nurses have skills in situations of conflict that drive them to seek out more information and understanding.

Two other groups of researchers suggest that the social worker is best prepared to use conflict management skills in the health care setting. Fandetti and Goldmeier argue that it is the role of the social worker in a health care setting to act as a mediator in those cases where there is a cultural conflict between the patient and the health care team. The authors maintain that social workers already play a mediating role in their work and that they are patient advocates.[40] Therefore, social workers are to facilitate the communication between the patient's cultural needs and the needs of the health care team. This requires a framework that the authors name "complexity of emergent ethnicity." The authors contend that social workers who are faced with a cultural conflict need to do an adequate assessment and implementation of the patient's situation. This means that the social worker must make an assessment on three levels: micro, mezzo and macro. The micro level is that of the individual patient's needs and desires. The mezzo level is the family, treatment teams and other subunits. The macro level is the hospital institution and the community. From this assessment the social worker would be in a position to adequately mediate a cultural conflict.

---

40. D. V. Fandetti and J. Goldmeier, "Social Workers as Culture Mediators in Health Care Settings," *Health and Social Work* 13, no. 3 (1988): 171-179. Social workers are sometimes referred to as "culture brokers," that is, as moving among cultures. A similar concept can be found for labour mediators, who are called "boundary spanners." For a description of boundary spanners, see R. A. Friedman and J. Podoiny, "Differentiation of Boundary Spanning Roles: Labor Negotiations and Implications for Role Conflict," *Administrative Science Quarterly* 37 (1992): 28-47.

Joseph and Conrad argue in a similar way.[41] Their article details a study on how social workers perceive their influence in ethical decision making in hospitals. The authors believe that as ethical decision making becomes more multidisciplinary in nature, social workers have the moral responsibility to respond to this changing situation. Yet ethical training is missing in most social workers' education. Consequently, social workers are not influential in ethical decision making in the hospitals. This goes contrary to the perceived role of the social worker as patient advocate. The authors, therefore, wanted to discover some of the necessary conditions for social workers' influence in ethical decision making in hospitals. They set out to make correlations among five independent variables: role clarity, role satisfaction, skill in information exchange, collaborative models of decision making and the effect of professional training in ethics. The dependent variable was the social worker's influence. This was operationalized as the social workers' "perception of their influence in the resolution of ethical conflict."[42] The authors made use of role theory because they believed that this theory was the foundation for other ethical frameworks (e.g., that of the American Hospital Association's report on ethical conflicts).[43]

Joseph and Conrad studied 123 master's students in social work. They used various questionnaires, most of which were developed for their study. This was primarily a correlational study. Their major findings suggest that the greater the clarity of the social worker's role and the greater his or her ability to share information, the greater the possibility that the social worker would be influential in ethical conflicts. Social workers also related better to a collaborative model of ethical decision making. The authors suggest that a course in professional ethics be taught to students at the master's level. This would provide the educational foundation necessary for the social worker's involvement in health care ethical deliberation.

---

41. M. V. Joseph and A. P. Conrad, "Social Work Influence on Interdisciplinary Ethical Decision Making in Health Care Settings," *Health and Social Work* 14, no. 1 (1989): 22-30. This article makes reference to the fact that often enough social workers do not feel competent in making contributions to ethical deliberations. This is in part due to their lack of ethical training. But it is also due to the problem of a conflict of professions. The role identity for social workers needs to emphasize that they are in equal status to other health care professionals. This can be addressed through the socialization of social workers (i.e., education).

42. Joseph and Conrad, "Social Work Influence," 25.

43. American Hospital Association, Special Committee on Biomedical Ethics, "Values in Conflict: Resolving Ethical Issues in Hospital Care," *American Hospital Association* (1985): 67-74.

CONFLICT RESOLUTION AND HOSPITAL ETHICS COMMITTEES

When health issues involve formal ethical dilemmas it sometimes falls to the hospital ethics committee to intervene.[44] Hundert argues that ethics committees need to follow a model of ethical deliberation.[45] This article is a presentation of his model. He borrows from John Rawls' concept of a "reflective equilibrium" to suggest that an ethics committee must balance out the competing values that are at stake in any particular ethical dilemma in order to arrive at a satisfactory resolution. The equilibrium would be reflective if the ethics committee represented the various viewpoints of the ethical dilemma. For example, one member may support patients' rights, while another may be concerned about financial limitations. These various perspectives would be kept in a dynamic tension through the balancing out of the perspectives within the ethics committee. Hundert claims his model allows the various values to be heard in the committee. Once understood by all members, there is the possibility that conflicts of value will dissolve through the options generated by the committee's dialogue. The aim of the model, therefore, is to structure the dialogue of the ethics committee in order to arrive at the best possible win-win solution. When an ethics committee has moved through this model a number of times it will establish a pattern of ethical deliberation that will be reflective of its members' moral principles. These moral principles are the equations of the worth of various incommensurable values. Unfortunately, Hundert is not clear about how his model actually controls the dialogue. For example, it is not clear how power imbalances might prohibit a reflective equilibrium. Fortunately, recent writers have addressed these issues more directly by making explicit use of conflict management skills and processes.

Maciunas and Moss discuss the role of ethics committees in cases where there is the necessity to determine whether the patient has the capacity

---

44. The distinction between formal and informal ethical dilemmas can be made by reference to the type of structure utilized to deliberate the dilemma. Formal structures include ethics committees, hospital boards and official regulatory bodies. Informal structures consist of private conversations, unilateral decisions and interventions by professional authorities (e.g., head nurse, attending physician and hospital administration). Most hospital ethical deliberation is of this kind.

45. E. Hundert, "A Model for Ethical Problem Solving in Medicine, with Practical Applications," *American Journal of Psychiatry* 144, no. 7 (1987): 839-846.

to make treatment decisions for him- or herself.[46] The authors claim that making this decision is the ethics committee's second most required task (the first is the withholding or withdrawing of life-sustaining treatments). The authors argue that the ethics committee's role is to facilitate the discourse among those involved in this kind of decision. They present a case study to describe their position.[47] In this particular case, the first responsibility of the ethics committee was to determine whether the patient had the capacity to make decisions about his treatment. They were able to affirm this question by carefully understanding the logic of the patient. The patient's logic was discovered through a comprehension of the situation as he saw it. In this case, the ethics committee facilitated a patient-care conference from which the authors "hoped that the patient and treating team would be able to negotiate a mutually acceptable plan."[48] This conference included the participation of the patient, his mother, the resident

---

46. K. A. Maciunas and A. H. Moss. "Learning the Patient's Narrative to Determine Decision-Making Capacity: The Role of Ethics Committees," *The Journal of Clinical Ethics* 3, no. 4 (1992): 287-289. This issue of *The Journal of Clinical Ethics* also contains two responses to the Maciunas and Moss article:

(1) Edward E. Waldron, "Ethics Committees, Decision-Making Quality Assurance, and Conflict Resolution," *The Journal of Clinical Ethics* 3, no. 4 (1992): 290-291. Waldron claims that the role of the ethics committee in determining decision-making quality assurance (DMQA) involves three questions: (1) Who should be involved in making the decision? (2) To what extent should each party be involved? and (3) Are all the members who need to be involved actually involved? In determining DMQA, the ethics committee must use active listening techniques such as learning the patient's story, because too often we only think that we understand what the other is saying. The key to an ethics committee is its flexibility. Facilitating decision making is an important additional role the ethics committee can contribute. In fact, Waldron writes, "if an ethics consultation service does nothing else, helping re-establish lines of communication between patient, family and care givers more than justifies its existence" (291).

(2) Mary B. West, "Mediation and Communication Techniques in Ethics Consultation," *The Journal of Clinical Ethics* 3, no. 4 (1992): 291-292. West concurs that the ethics committee, when making an ethical consultation, must use facilitation techniques that attempt to understand the patient's point of view and his or her underlying interest, fears and needs. The ethics consultation must understand the patient's internal logic. Yet different ethical consultations depend upon other conditions. West concludes, "the most appropriate process for an ethics committee or consultation depends on the nature of the issue, the parties involved, the committee's role in the institution and the goals for that consultation" (292). For example, in the case presented in the Maciunas and Moss article, the ethics committee had two goals: first, to determine the decision-making capacity of the patient and, second, to facilitate the discussion on the best treatment.

47. Maciunas and Moss, "Learning the Patient's Narrative." This case involved a middle-aged patient with some cognitive processing difficulties. He refused further treatment against the advice of his doctors and his mother.

48. Ibid., 288.

physician, the primary nurse and the social worker. The authors write that the ethics committee has four roles to fulfil. First, it must learn the patient's story. No treatment plan can be acceptable without a complete understanding of the patient's perspective. Second, it must facilitate communication among the health care team, family and patient. This helps to create the necessary trust among the participants in an open and mutual exchange for effective problem solving. Third, the ethics committee will have to be the patient's advocate. Fourth, the ethics committee fulfils the requirement of a third-party mediator by assisting with various conflict resolution techniques. Unfortunately, the article does not detail how this facilitation went about in their case study.

West and McIver Gibson describe the specific use of conflict management processes within the ethics committee in order to resolve the different kinds of problems these committees face. Their article is a summary of a project sponsored by the National Institute for Dispute Resolution and the University of New Mexico.[49] The study's aim was to understand how ethics committees view their roles and how they go about their work. The study also looked at how mediation/facilitation could augment the ethics committee role and internal process.

The article begins by describing the conflict resolution spectrum of structures—from negotiation to litigation. The authors make the following distinction between mediation and facilitation: mediation refers to third-party intervention of defined disputes; facilitation refers to intervention without a defined dispute. Based on this distinction, the authors describe the stages of mediation: intake, introduction and contracting, information gathering and issue identification, agenda setting and reaching resolution, agreement writing and follow-up. The processes of mediation and facilitation make use of such techniques as passive and active listening. Passive listening refers to the use of silence and noncommittal nodding. Active listening refers to techniques aimed at establishing understanding among the disputants. These techniques especially help to balance power.

Not all hospital ethics committees, however, are alike. There is a wide discrepancy in their role and function. Whether alternative dispute resolution process "will be effective for medical ethics committees necessarily depends on the roles and functions those committees fulfil in their institutions."[50] All the committees surveyed were interdisciplinary.

---

49. M. B. West and J. McIver Gibson, "Facilitating Medical Ethics Case Review: What Ethics Committees Can Learn from Mediation and Facilitation Techniques," *Cambridge Quarterly on Healthcare Ethics* 1 (1992): 63-74.

50. West and McIver Gibson, "Facilitating Medical Ethics Case Review," 65-66.

Each thought their role to be nonintrusive and believed that the parties involved, not the committee, should make the final decision. Most committees viewed their role as educator. The makeup of the committees differed among those of exclusive membership, limited membership or inclusive membership. "Committee composition appears to reflect committees' views of their roles in their institutions."[51] Education roles were inclusive in membership. Problem-solving roles were exclusive in membership.

"A committee's source of power affected how the committee views its institutional role."[52] From the work of Mayer, the authors describe ten sources of power. The authors contend that the personal power of the ethicist is an important consideration in the ethics committee. The significant sources of power must be considered in the committee. "The pervasive imbalance of power among participants such as patients, families, nurses, physicians and lawyers is a critical consideration in case consultations."[53] Power distribution may reflect the role a committee plays in the institution. A committee that sees its role as educational will likely have a more balanced power distribution.

The form and process of the ethics committee differed widely across the committees studied. This is in some way reflective of the committee's role in the institution, dominant members' perspectives and historical practice. Usually, ethics committees do not refer to ethical dilemmas as conflicts or disputes. "The content of consultations most often involves interdisciplinary concerns (legal, religious and sometimes economic) and end-of-life issues such as life-support treatment decisions and 'medically futile' treatment."[54] Ethics committees gave little attention to their own process. This raised three concerns: (1) How does the committee conduct meetings? (2) How do members see their role within their institution? (3) How do they conduct case consultations? Ethics committees use some form of shuttle facilitation, mediation and large group facilitation.[55]

The authors make three recommendations. First, ethics committees need better intake procedures. They recommend that someone be trained in mediation intake procedures to properly establish the process among the participants. This can help set up the process and at times resolve certain problems before they reach the committee. Second, the model of case consultation should vary according to the committee's role, the nature

---

51. Ibid., 66.

52. Ibid., 66.

53. Ibid., 67.

54. Ibid., 68.

55. Ibid., 69-70.

of the issue and the parties involved. Three primary processes were developed that could be correlated with committee role: issue resolution, issue exploration and education. Third, the ethics committee should have an established follow-up procedure. This will provide information to the committee on the outcomes of their work and will further avail them to the ongoing relations among the participants.

The authors conclude that the use of mediation and facilitation is dependent upon these variables: role of the committee, committee power, types of cases and committee's goal in consultation. It is clear that mediation and facilitation will augment the work of the committee under these considerations.

A COLLABORATIVE MODEL FOR HEALTH CARE PROFESSIONALS

The use of conflict management techniques and process in the health care setting need not be limited to the formal ethics committee. Changing professional roles of health care workers demand that a more collaborative model of intervention be established as the structure for their professional interactions. Hayes, Soniat and Burr[56] describe a model of collaborative ethical decision making by taking up the case of forcing services on older adults who are "at risk" of personal harm. This model asks four sets of questions: (1) What are the professional and personal value differences? Are these clarified for everyone? (2) How are these different perspectives integrated into a collaborative team decision about treatment? Is one perspective dominant, or is equality sought? (3) Who is ultimately responsible for the decision? (4) How are dissenting or minority voices registered? These authors maintain that these questions are not usually raised in case conferences. Their model attempts to make these questions deliberate and open for all the participants. This will increase the collaborative arrangement among the professionals since all are included in the deliberation. This participation should also increase the sense of responsibility, thereby reducing the likelihood that any one professional will hinder the outcome of the team decision. The authors believe that "extracting and directly confronting value differences can facilitate communication between disciplines and individual team members."[57] Although consensus may not always be reached, this model nevertheless proposes

---

56. C. L. Hayes, B. Soniat and H. Burr, "Value Conflict and Resolution in Forcing Services on 'At Risk' Community-Based Older Adults," *Clinical Gerontologist* 4, no. 3 (1986): 41-48.

57. Hayes, Soniat and Burr, "Value Conflict," 47.

"a multi-disciplinary approach and encourages explicit statements of values, discussion of professional ethics, and sharing of perceptions and judgments among professional disciplines."[58]

Other authors have also urged for the use of conflict management within specific health care settings. For example, Gralnick[59] suggests that the resolution of professional conflict is constitutive of quality care for psychiatric patients. The treatment of patients in mental health facilities usually requires a broad range of therapeutic procedures (medical and nonmedical, individual and group). These procedures are meant to help the patient work out resolutions of his or her internal differences. Within a hospital therapeutic setting this working out is done within the social unit of the hospital comprised of patients and staff. This therapeutic community is prone to a number of different kinds of conflict. There are conflicts among staff, among patients and among staff and patients. Gralnick argues, therefore, that the resolution of these various conflicts is a crucial part of therapy. Gralnick lists a number of qualifications that the personnel of the mental health hospital would have to possess in order to adequately meet the challenge of resolving conflicts that emerge in their context. Part of these qualifications is a commitment to fostering an environment for the potential growth of a patient. Such an environment would foster trust among the participants. Those involved should be convinced of the role that the resolution of conflicts plays in the overall therapeutic process of the patients. This is important because the hospital is a social setting with its own set of values. The patient, who previous to admittance lived his or her own set of values, must now adapt to the system of the hospital. In this adaptation conflicts of values arise. The ongoing resolution of these conflicts is essential to the health of the patient. Gralnick describes two examples. In these examples it is clear that the conflicts that are described interfered in the daily life of the patients and the staff. Through deliberate and open communication there was the attempt to reach a consensus and resolve the conflict. At all times the issues of the conflicts were brought into the actual therapeutic relationship as part of the patient's overall therapy. In the resolution of these conflicts there emerged more common understanding of the hospital's values and goals among all the participants. This understanding creates the necessary trust of the therapeutic environment. Such trust is essential for the ongoing growth of every patient. Thus, in a hospital setting, where there exists a multiple arrangement of relationships among staff and patient, the resolution of

---

58. Ibid., 47.

59. A. Gralnick, "Conflict Resolution and Inhospital Therapeutic Process," *Psychiatric Journal of the University of Ottawa* 12, no. 1 (1987): 21-25.

the multilevel conflicts becomes a critical component of the therapeutic process, if not the very process itself.[60]

From a nursing perspective, Pike advocates for a collaborative model of ethical decision making among health care professionals. In her article, Pike describes a collaborative intensive care unit at Beth Israel Hospital in Boston.[61] Pike argues that nurses' moral outrage at difficult ethical decisions can be reduced if there is a collaborative effort among the health care professionals by making ethical deliberations together. The outrage nurses feel is conditioned by internal and external factors. Internal factors are those such as a nurse's lack of professional ethical training and confidence. External factors include the authority of physicians, hospital policy and legal positions of professionals. A collaborative model, however, promotes "shared decision making, responsibility, and accountability [that] effectively dismantles some of the most prominent internal and external constraints."[62] This collaboration is based upon three factors. First, all the professionals openly acknowledge that they share the common goal of the health and comfort of the patient. Second, health care providers work not as autonomous professionals, but within an interdependent relationship. Everyone shares in the responsibility and accountability for the level of care offered to their patients. Third, their working together is meant to build trust, respect and understanding. There must be acknowledged a concerned effort to address conflict at its source rather than let it escalate. There is also "associated with this acknowledgement [the] appreciation of all perspectives in decision making and a commitment to come to the negotiation process

---

60. Gralnick, "Conflict Resolution," 25. Gralnick does not address, however, the possibility that in the event of the resolution of the conflict of value between the patient's value system and the value system of the hospital, the value system of the hospital would be altered as well as the value system of the patient. For Gralnick, the value system of the hospital is designed by the professionals with some input by the patients, but "it may not be said that they (the patients) play a major part" (22). Since the staff is more rational, argues Gralnick, it is they who determine right from wrong and acceptable behaviour from unacceptable behaviour. One is left to wonder, however, whether the resolution of these value conflicts is in fact the accommodation to the hospital's value system on the part of the patient, rather than a resolution that challenges *both* systems of value.

61. Pike, "Moral Outrage." Karl Slaikeu, "Designing Dispute Resolution Systems in the Health Care Industry," *Negotiation Journal* 5, no. 4 (1989): 395-400, describes his initiatives at integrating conflict management skills and processes throughout the personnel structure of a hospital. This involved, for example, training staff members in conflict management skills and providing both formal and informal mediation structures within the hospital institution. Unfortunately, Slaikeu does not mention whether such processes were used for the deliberation of ethical disputes.

62. Pike, "Moral Outrage," 352.

with an open mind."[63] This will naturally change the way professionals view each other in their working relationship. Power and authority configurations shift as everyone acknowledges the input of other professionals.[64] There exists, therefore, a common base upon which health care providers can deliver their care.[65] Pike calls this common base "synergy." This synergy is not just cooperation. It is a combination of the various professional perspectives into a common perspective.[66] For example, it allows the blending of moral perspectives from both male (as justice-oriented) and female (as care-oriented) advantages. Pike writes that "a collaborative alliance seems to allow for the merger of these levels in such a way that, in the end, a higher level is reached."[67] This higher level is a more comprehensive viewpoint of the medical/ethical situation. It involves the perspectives of the professionals and the patient. In fact, this synergy, or collaborative model, facilitates moral discourse across both

---

63. Ibid., 353.

64. The issue of power in the physician–nurse relationship has been addressed from a feminist theological perspective by H. J. Schattschneider, "Power Relationships Between Physician and Nurse," *Humane Medicine* 6, no. 3 (1990): 197-201. Schattschneider challenges the traditional physician–nurse relationship as promoting inequality. Her feminist theological perspective offers an "ethics of liberation" from this traditional power inequality in search of a relationship that promotes equality, balance of power, mutual trust and respect.

65. The idea that these professionals need a common basis of shared meaning is also expressed by D. Gibson, "Theory and Strategies for Resolving Conflict," *Occupational Therapy in Mental Health* 5, no. 4 (1986): 47-64. Gibson writes, "members of groups who show allegiance to superordinate organizational goals, who share mutually facilitating interests, and who are bonded to common values or a common community are likely to resolve issues more cooperatively than those without such bonds" (54). The structure of conflict management processes promotes the development of these shared bonds of meaning throughout the life of the multidisciplinary, professional team.

66. A study by R. M. Walker, S. H. Miles, C. B. Stocking and M. Siegler, "Physicians' and Nurses' Perceptions of Ethics Problems on General Medical Services," *Journal of General Intern Medicine* 6 (1991): 424-429, suggests that the level of professional ethical conflict is associated with the different perspectives of the nurse and the doctor based upon: (1) their different understandings of their professional tasks; (2) professional discord (e.g., nurses tended to focus upon physician errors); and (3) difference in professional orientation of what is considered an ethical problem. These authors suggest that physicians and nurses need a joint educational program that would have "the advantage of allowing a direct and personal sharing of perspectives without the restraining influence of real or perceived discrepancies in power and authority. Such an approach, coupled with joint training in collaborative care, conflict management, and communication skills, might prepare physicians and nurses to deal more openly and directly with issues of clinical ethics" (429).

67. Pike, "Moral Outrage," 360.

patient and professional perspectives. Although it may not always reach consensus, it does "put an end to the fighting, manipulation, avoidance, deceit and power struggles that have been so characteristic of moral conflicts in the patient care arena."[68]

This section surveyed some initiatives promoting conflict management techniques and processes within the health care setting. The demand for conflict management skills and process will increase as professional relationships change, as ethics committees become more influential within hospitals and as a more collaborative model of professional interaction takes place within the hospital setting. These skills and processes will be used in order to manage multilevel conflicts, including ethical dilemmas, treatment plans and interstaff disputes. This does not mean that the business of caring for people will become any easier. In fact, conflict management processes may require more time and more effort than traditional methods of resolving disputes. The integration of these processes, however, is made with the hope that the health care environment among professionals will become mutual, open, trusting and equal. It is within an environment with such values as these that better care will be provided.

---

68. Ibid., 358.

Conclusion to Part 2

Kenneth R. Melchin

Part 2 of this project began with a survey of literature in the field of discourse ethics. Chapter 6, by James Sauer, identified two main lines of theory in this field—the proceduralists and the contextualists—and provided preliminary arguments for the complementarity of the two. Chapter 7, by Kenneth R. Melchin, introduced the cognitional theory of Bernard Lonergan as an ethical framework for the project and drew upon insights from Lonergan scholarship to identify how proceduralists, contextualists and cognitional theorists can contribute to an understanding of ethical discourse in health care teams. The work of part 1 of the project— the analysis of implicit ethics of health care professionals—was identified as a contribution to contextualist analysis. The field of conflict resolution was identified as providing resources for a proceduralist analysis of ethical discourse. Finally, chapter 8, by Peter Monette, surveyed extant literature in conflict resolution to specify some of these contributions, to situate them within the ethical theory framework and to draw out theoretical and practical implications for ethical discourse in health care teams.

The conclusion of this stage of the research is that, contrary to the expectations of contextualist and proceduralist theorists, neither of these bodies of theory on their own will yield complete sets of principles for the resolution of all aspects of value conflicts. Rather, value conflicts are only resolved by communities of men and women implementing the cognitional operations and skills of experience, understanding, judgment and decision in ethical discourse. Furthermore, the cognitional structure analysis of Lonergan, on its own, does not yield immediate solutions to value conflicts. Cognitional theory provides insights into the four levels of operations. It remains for women and men to draw upon the fruits of the contextualist and proceduralist analyses within a framework provided by an appropriation of the four levels of operations of ethical deliberation in concrete instances of ethical deliberation.

What we did find is that understanding the four levels of cognitional operations provides helpful tools for identifying, evaluating and integrating the diverse contributions of participants in the ethical deliberation process. In much discourse, the values that shape participants' handling of cases are often first-level values, positions and desires that reflect an individual's experience of the situation. However, a more careful scrutiny of these first-level reactions to cases often reveals the presence of deeper, more complex feelings, convictions, interests and responsibilities that reflect the participant's vision of the wider context of social order in which the case fits. Often, when these implicit ideas and convictions about social order are raised to explicit awareness, they express a professional's sense of responsibility toward persons and institutions. Understanding and articulating these deeper values makes it possible to reflect on them, to evaluate them, to subject them to critical scrutiny in the light of the experiences and insights of others. This third level of operations seeks to raise and answer all of the relevant questions so that participants can make judgments about the best direction for programs of care. Finally, the commitment to implement the programs of care makes it possible for participants to work out and take responsibility for strategies of action that will coordinate the diverse contributions of professionals into common projects toward the well-being of clients and patients.

We found an interesting correlation between the findings from the field of conflict studies and the fourfold structure of ethical deliberation. Conflict researchers place considerable emphasis on the task of explicitly articulating implicit feelings and convictions in the discourse process. Conflicts are often driven by implicit concerns that lie behind explicit positions and, as long as the discourse stays focussed on the positions, the deeper issues seldom get resolved. Researchers have shown that participants need to move through an opening stage where they articulate their first-level positions, but they also need to move to a second stage where they probe beyond the positions for these underlying concerns. This process includes recognizing and validating the concerns of others so that, in a third stage, common underlying concerns can be articulated. This common ground creates a platform or framework for the participants to move forward together to work out programs of action. This four-stage process seems to reflect Lonergan's cognitional levels and provides participants in team deliberations with tools for moving through the discourse process, attentive to the diverse contributions of others while on the lookout for common frameworks for working through differences.

Research on conflict resolution in health care reflects a wide range of efforts to implement some of these insights in practice. Furthermore, this research also reveals an attention to professionals and professional styles in the deliberation process. The insights from this part of the study offer a conceptual framework for understanding these diverse contributions and linking them together into an integrative vision.

The implication for the next stage of the research is that the understanding and responsible management of ethical discourse need to draw upon all of these diverse lines of research. Criteria for moving through the four levels of ethical meaning in the deliberations can be drawn from Lonergan's cognitional theory. Criteria for analyzing the way in which the social and institutional contexts of health care professionals are implicated in cases can be drawn from the study in part 1 of the implicit ethics of professionals in health care teams. Finally, criteria for understanding and managing the structural dynamics of the discourse itself can be drawn from the essays surveying research results in the field of conflict resolution.

In part 3 of this project, researchers draw upon the insights of these three diverse fields to make a series of observations on simulated cases of ethical discourse involving health care professionals in the field of pediatric chronic care. Since the goals of the project are both theoretical and practical, we take the final step of constructing a practical guide to help professionals in their ethical deliberations.

PART 3

**ACTION RESEARCH:
ETHICAL DELIBERATION
IN MULTIPROFESSIONAL
HEALTH CARE TEAMS**

Introduction to Part 3

Kenneth R. Melchin

Part 3 of this study takes the results of parts 1 and 2 and applies them to a case-study, action-research context. Two teams of health care professionals from Anglophone and Francophone pediatric chronic care institutional settings volunteered to participate in videotaped discussions of case studies involving ethical issues typically encountered in their work. These videos were then examined by the research team in the light of the analyses of parts 1 and 2. In keeping with the overall goals of this study, the observers focussed on the ethical deliberation process. We sought to determine whether insights from the implicit ethics of professionals and insights from conflict studies and ethical theory could help understand the dynamics of the deliberation process and help practitioners in their efforts to wrestle with the issues.

Chapter 9, "Action Research on Ethical Deliberation," presents a summary discussion of the results of the action research part of this project and is written by Kenneth R. Melchin and Peter Monette. The observations and insights presented here were developed through the course of a long series of discussions among the members of the research team: Peter Monette, Tim Flaherty, Jean-Marc Larouche, Hubert Doucet, Kevin G. Murphy and Kenneth R. Melchin. In addition, they represent a distillation and summary of a large body of notes and anecdotal observations taken from repeated instances of viewing the videotaped deliberation sessions. They do not attempt to offer exhaustive analyses of the data, nor do they claim to offer statistical methods and controls in support of the conclusions. These goals would have fallen well beyond the limits of what reasonably could have been attempted in the project. Rather, the effort here has been to do an initial "road test" of some of the theoretical insights from parts 1 and 2 of the project and to present the results of this effort in a summary discussion. The goal is to suggest a line of analysis that could be carried further and substantiated more firmly in subsequent research.

Chapter 10 presents the *Guide for Ethical Deliberation*. The action research of the project was conducted in two stages, with two sets of videotaped deliberation sessions. After the first set of sessions, the research team drew upon the results of the work of part 1 and our observations of the first round of sessions to construct a guide to help the various professionals in health care teams become attentive to the ethical deliberation process and to their own form of participation in the process. Emphasis in developing the guide was on simplicity and accessibility. We sought, as much as possible, to provide a tool that would draw on technical multidisciplinary research but would still be of service to professionals unfamiliar with the technical languages of the diverse disciplines.

Chapter 11, "Thinking About Ethical Deliberation in Multiprofessional Health Care Teams," offers an opportunity to stand back and reflect on the whole project. It presents some indications as to how the various parts fit together to complement and enrich each other. This study has moved forward on a number of fronts, engaging diverse bodies of theoretical and practically oriented research. Part 1 began with an extensive literature analysis on the implicit ethics of health care professionals and concluded with a range of "types," each with their own implied value judgments about the goals and tasks of their profession and the form of interaction with other professionals. Part 2 ranged through literature on ethical theory and conflict studies to draw out some theoretical tools for the analysis of the ethical deliberation process. Part 3 has sought to provide concrete opportunities for testing some of these ideas in action. And we have proposed a framework, drawn from the work of Lonergan, for understanding how the contributions from these diverse fields of analysis can come together in an integrative vision. This chapter tries to pull these pieces together to see how the whole process "works." It concludes by suggesting lines of further research that could build upon and provide empirical testing of the hypotheses formulated here. The text is written by Kenneth R. Melchin but, again, the ideas come from long sessions of discussions among the members of the research team.

Chapter 9

Action Research on Ethical Deliberation

Kenneth R. Melchin
and Peter Monette

The goals of this action-research stage of the project were twofold: (1) to determine, on the basis of an anecdotal study of the videos, if evidence of the features of ethical deliberation in multiprofessional teams gleaned from the analyses of parts 1 and 2 could be observed in the case conferences; (2) to use insights from the literature and observations from the videos to construct a *Guide for Ethical Deliberation* that could aid health care professionals in their ethical deliberations.

The work of the action research went forward with these two goals pursued concurrently. The members of the research team, Peter Monette, Tim Flaherty and Kevin G. Murphy, under the direction of Kenneth R. Melchin, Jean-Marc Larouche and Hubert Doucet, began by conducting the background research for the case conference sessions, writing four case studies involving ethical issues typically encountered in pediatric chronic care and constructing the analytical grid of questions from parts 1 and 2 of the project. The analytical grid used in studying the deliberation sessions was prepared by Peter Monette and Tim Flaherty and is presented in appendix B. The case studies were prepared by Kevin G. Murphy under the direction of Hubert Doucet and are presented in appendix C of this volume.

Arrangements were made for two sets of staged ethical deliberation sessions involving two teams of health care professionals. This was coordinated by Hubert Doucet. While the deliberations deal with prepared cases, the participants ensured that the discussions were representative of the sorts of sessions that typically arise in real-life contexts. The deliberation sessions of the first series were one-hour long and conducted in French, and each was devoted to the discussion of one case. The sessions were videotaped by the research team. As the tapes came in, they were examined by the team, first for preliminary anecdotal observations without explicit use of the analytical grid and, second, for more detailed case-study observations, using the grid.

As the analysis of this first set of deliberation sessions proceeded, the research team began compiling notes and preparing a draft of the *Guide for Ethical Deliberation*. The final version of the guide is presented in chapter 10 of this volume. Arrangements were made for a second set of deliberation sessions involving an English-speaking health care team. The team members were given the guide and were asked to attempt a preliminary implementation of the guide in their deliberations. As the videos from these sessions came in, researchers studied them and made anecdotal observations, again using the three-part analytical grid.

The project uses an action-research approach. This methodology is an adaptation of the social analysis method of Holland and Henriot and the *recherche-action* method of Grand'Maison.[1] This method was chosen because of its explicit concern with values, social structures and practical action.[2] In addition, because the method does not focus on quantitative verification of existing hypotheses within the context of extant theory, it permits an anecdotal case-study analysis to draw upon multiple theories and disciplines to contribute to the development of new insights, new theory and recommendations for practical action. By using a combination of literature review, multidisciplinary theoretical analysis and anecdotal case analysis, this project aims at developing theoretical and practical tools that could be subjected to more empirically rigorous scrutiny in future research projects.

---

1. See Joe Holland and Peter Henriot, *Social Analysis*, rev. ed. (Maryknoll, N.Y.: Orbis/ Center of Concern, 1984); Jacques Grand'Maison and Solange Lefebvre, eds., *Une génération bouc émissaires: Enquête sur les baby boomers*, 3ᵉ dossier de la recherche-action dans le diocèse Saint-Jérôme (Montreal: Fides, 1993); Jacques Grand'Maison and Solange Lefebvre, eds., *La Part des aînées: Recherche-action*, 4ᵉ dossier (Montreal: Fides, 1994); Jean-Guy Nadeau, ed., *La Praxéologie pastorale: Orientations et parcours*, vols. 1 and 2. *Cahiers d'études pastorales IV* (Montreal: Fides, 1987); *Colloque recherche action*, Actes du Colloque recherche action, Université du Québec à Chicoutimi, 1981 (Chicoutimi: Université du Québec à Chicoutimi, 1982); J. Billiet et al., *Actes du colloque: Méthodologie et pratique de la recherche-action* (Brussels: Royaume de Belgique, Programme national de recherche en sciences sociales, 1980).

2. See Holland and Henriot, 98-100. One modification of the Holland–Henriot methodology involved the range of "root metaphors" informing the understanding of the social structures implicated in health care. Holland and Henriot draw upon Gibson Winter, *Liberating Creation* (New York: Crossroad, 1981), for an artistic "root metaphor" to guide their analysis. Consequently, their work has a "liberation" or "critique of domination" focus to it and, therefore, tends to look for the unjust or oppressive tendencies of social order. However, in his earlier work *Elements for a Social Ethic* (New York: Macmillan, 1966), Winter outlined three different metaphors of sociality, each with its own potential realm of application to society. Two of these, the behaviourist and the functionalist, embrace a more sympathetic view of social order. This work recognizes a more comprehensive range of potential "root metaphors" operative in the diverse professional styles and in the diverse forms of social structures relevant to ethical discourse in health care settings.

The cases deal with ethical issues in pediatric chronic care, however *the focus of this project is on the process of ethical deliberation in multiprofessional health care teams.* Consequently, while research for the cases involved considerable study of the ethical issues themselves and while the concern of the health care professionals was with the issues, the discussions and analyses in the pages that follow focus on the deliberation process itself. The research seeks to advance the understanding of ethical deliberation and to develop tools to aid professionals in this process. In chapter 11 we offer some reflections on the links between the issues and the process. The assumption is that ethical understanding is advanced by health care professionals who wrestle with issues in their work experience and that tools to help the team deliberation process can enrich reflection on the issues.

The discussions of the observations of the action research team are grouped into three subsections: "Implicit Ethics of Professionals," "Deliberation Process" and "Ethical Structure." Using the questions of the analytical grid, the team members sought to identify the constructive and dysfunctional features of the deliberation process that came into focus when viewed against the backdrop of the work of parts 1 and 2 of the project.

IMPLICIT ETHICS OF PROFESSIONALS

Generally, the deliberations of the health care professionals revealed evidence of a diversity of professional types. In addition, all of the cases involved participants who showed evidence of more than one professional type. However, when discussion became more lively, there seemed to be a tendency for participants to revert to a particular type, perhaps the type most familiar to them. Generally, what distinguished the types were the observable evidence of the implicit value concerns that characterized their forms of professional commitment.

Physicians tended to fall into the Expert and Team Leader types with their respective concerns with: (1) scientific data and institutional-authority-based decision making; and (2) consultative decision making. With a few exceptions (the notable examples of the nurse Managers), nurses tended to fall into the Advocate and Coordinator types with their respective commitments to: (1) the dignity of the child; and (2) collaboration with child and family. On occasion, nurses showed evidence of the Manager type with their concern for codes of action and institutions. Social workers generally revealed a commitment to the integration of child, family and community interests, typical of their professional type. At times, participants showed evidence of interprofessional and intraprofessional alliances between professional types. In such cases, the expressed concerns of one professional were sometimes met with confirmation by another. At other times, conflicting types resulted in open discussion over the relevance of one or another expressed value-aspect of the case.

Overall, the participants seemed to engage in the deliberation animated by their implicit commitments to the ethical objectives of their various professional types as they seemed relevant to the case and the discourse at the time. The effect of their implicit ethical convictions seemed to be to highlight the relevance of those aspects of the case that related to their assumed professional obligations. As these aspects of the case became apparent, participants articulated them openly in the discourse. When discussion followed upon their interventions, these aspects of the case were assessed openly by the group in relation to the other aspects articulated by others.

Throughout the case conferences, the health care teams did not often use explicitly ethical language nor did they appear to engage in what they explicitly understood to be ethical deliberation. However, the ethical commitments implicit to their various professional types still tended to direct their discourse toward ethically relevant aspects of the case. To the degree that these aspects were responded to by others, discussed, explored and evaluated in the discourse of the team, the ethical concerns as understood through professional commitment shaped the eventual outcomes, even when the team devoted no explicit attention to the issues as ethical. To the degree that implicit value concerns were brought to light in the deliberations but not responded to or assessed by the team, these ethical aspects of the case did not tend to shape the outcomes.

The diversity of professional value concerns among members of the teams had the effect that a wide range of ethically relevant data was brought into the open discourse. When cases are complex, as these were, this diversity is an important feature of ethical deliberation. In general, professionals deal with different aspects or dimensions of the lives of their clients. When they understand their professional commitments differently, they tend to focus attention on different aspects of their clients' relations with family, community, culture, health care professionals and institutions. All of these relations bring diverse ranges of ethically relevant data into the discourse.

When alliances among professions arose, expressed value concerns were restated, discussed openly by others and, at times, assessed and weighed in relation to other value concerns. In addition, observable alliances had the effect of adding weight or legitimacy to value-aspects of the case, which previously may not have been recognized as important by the group. When conflicts among types resulted in open conflictual discourse among professionals, participants tended to assess, weigh, evaluate and argue conflicting concerns in relation to wider aspects of the case. Consequently, diversity of professional types, alliances and conflicts tended to have the constructive effect of bringing diverse value-aspects of a case to light and subjecting them to open, multiparty scrutiny in health care discourse. This remained so even when the discourse did not make explicit appeal to ethical language and analytic tools.

I have been summarizing the *constructive* features of the deliberation among professionals. Generally, the implicit ethical commitments of diverse professional types tended to direct participants' attention toward a variety of value-aspects of a case and to bring these value-aspects into open discussion and analysis in the deliberation process. The *dysfunctional* features of the professional types pertained to the way in which forms of professional interaction tended to hamper the articulation, elaboration and evaluation of these value concerns.

One of the more prevalent forms of dysfunctional interaction observed by the researchers concerned professional hierarchies, power imbalances and dominance among professional types. Researchers observed that leadership in the case discussions was often taken by the Expert or Manager types of physicians or nurses. The effect here was that the implicit value concerns of these professional types tended to focus and direct the group's discussion. When this dominance was strong, discussion of these particular value concerns tended to monopolize the case conferences.

In a number of cases, there seemed to be a tendency of some professionals to defer to others, perhaps to their authority, whether personal or institutional, thus adding weight or legitimacy to some value-aspects of the case. At times this seemed to correlate with nonparticipation of some professionals. At other times, the expressed concerns of other professionals received little or no attention or follow-up in the deliberation process.

Researchers observed that in the opening stages of some case conferences, a physician's presentation of the medical or physiological aspects of a case often set the tone and direction of the group's discussion of the case. While this opening "narrative" had the effect of articulating a range of value-aspects of the case, it also had the effect of inviting subsequent interventions relating to the medical or physiological value-aspects of the case and discouraging others. In these instances, the opening narrative appeared to act as an implicit criterion of relevance for the value-aspects of the case that would be invited or admitted into the deliberation process.

Another point in the discourse where the influence of professional hierarchy and dominance was observable was in the formulation of action strategies. Researchers observed moments when professionals with a more senior institutional status, usually physicians, formulated action strategies and others accepted them or recommended them for implementation without significant discussion. At times, these professionals were designated to implement the strategies. Again, if professional status has the effect of influencing the evaluation of action strategies, then the other value concerns of other professional types will not be allowed to exercise their critical modulating effect in the discourse.

One of the difficulties that come to light in this discussion of the dysfunctional effects of professional interactions pertains to the difference between implicit and explicit ethics. In large measure, the value-aspects of the case that were observed in the research were not formulated in explicitly ethical language by the health care professionals. Rather, they were communicated implicitly by them. Explicitly, the participants tended to focus on the events, actions, clinical data of the case, strategies for action and specific consequences of proposed programs of care. Participants did not often probe beyond these case-specific details to explicitly analyze their implications for professional obligations, institutional responsibilities, public rights and goods or more generalized notions of justice or value. Researchers were able to identify the interventions of the participants as, in fact, value-aspects of the case, not because the participants articulated them as such, but because they implicitly revealed features of professional ethos that were identified in the literature.

In some instances, this lack of explicit ethical reflection seemed to pose no significant problems. However, problems seemed to occur when important ethical conflicts arose in a case and when professionals continued to deal with the issues implicitly in terms of the professional commitments specific to their own professional type or types. In these moments, the value conflicts seemed vulnerable to being influenced by professional hierarchy and authority relations.

As long as ethics were implicit, the diverse and conflicting ethical aspects of a case tended to remain vulnerable to being dealt with through the forms of personal and professional interaction among members of the team rather than through critical ethical analysis. If dominant figures championed physiology values, discussion tended to focus on these values, often excluding or downplaying the importance of other ethically relevant data such as home or community relationships, health care institutional obligations or religious commitments. Without attending explicitly to the issues as ethical, health care practitioners had no way of subjecting the value-aspects of the case to explicit ethical judgment and the tendency was for the typical patterns of professional authority relations operative among team members to shape the resolution of the value conflicts.

One final note. It may be the case that in certain health care institutional settings, certain forms of hierarchy and authority relations may be appropriate. However, in ethical discourse, these authority relations cannot be allowed to exert a controlling influence. What is important here is the role that diverse professional types have in bringing to light and enabling others to appreciate diverse value-aspects of cases. As long as professionals of a variety of types participate fully in ethical discourse, all team members will have the opportunity to attend to value-aspects of the case that they might tend to overlook and all must wrestle with weighing and assessing the significance of these diverse aspects in formulating action strategies.[3]

DELIBERATION PROCESS

The main constructive feature of the deliberation process observed in the case conferences that reflected the literature in conflict resolution involved the articulation of diverse positions by participants. Quite a number of diverse positions were observed throughout the cases. Positions are distinguishable from underlying concerns by their specificity and their reference to particular actions and concrete goals that individuals desire to achieve. Underlying concerns, on the other hand, point toward broader, more wide-ranging concerns that bear upon multiple aspects and dimensions of social living. Generally, many of the diverse positions are articulated in the opening stages of the deliberation process. However, this is by no means exclusively the case.

Positions were often articulated when participants gained entry into the discourse. In some cases researchers observed that participants had ample opportunity to speak. In a debriefing session, one participant made reference to these opportunities and observed that a colleague made an explicit effort to solicit the input of all, with noticeable positive effects.

One other observable discourse-structure feature was the occasional effort to probe beyond positions to underlying concerns. In a number of cases some probing was noticeable. In one instance, this probing had an observable effect on changing the action strategy. In general, however, this probing was infrequent.

A number of discourse skill features were observed. In four cases there were some observable efforts to clarify the meanings of others. In one case there was evidence of clarifying and restating. And in another case one participant's efforts to summarize had the effect of moving the group to a reassessment of their action strategy.

---

3.   The argument here is that different spheres of action call for different forms of ethical obligations, particularly obligations concerning work relations and discourse relations among professionals. It is the structure of social action in the particular sphere of life that sets the ground for the form of the ethical obligations. For a similar argument relating the obligations of justice to diverse spheres of social life, see Michael Walzer, *Spheres of Justice* (New York: Basic Books, 1983).

What was most noticeable about the case conferences was the relative lack of overt conflict and the conspicuous ease with which participants arrived at consensus on action strategies. While the potentially problematic aspects of this feature will be discussed below, it is important to observe here that participants in the case conferences showed considerable respect toward each other, a willingness to work with each other, a concern to move quickly toward action and a common commitment to finding a consensus on strategies for action. Consensus on action strategies often emerged quickly in the discussions. In all likelihood, the time limits of the discourse sessions would have had the effect of adding a note of urgency and a preoccupation with action to their deliberations. Indeed, such time constraints probably affect most of their real-life professional deliberations.

Still, there remained a number of *dysfunctional* features that could be observed in the deliberations. The following discussion of dysfunctional features of the discourse structure, based as it is upon literature in the field of conflict resolution, focusses on features that create, sustain or exacerbate conflicts. It might be argued that this literature is hardly relevant to these case conferences since the discourse sessions revealed little evidence of overt conflict. Indeed, this argument has some validity. Conflict literature is, in large measure, devoted to diagnosing problematic features in the structure of discourse that are causing conflicts or creating obstacles to resolution. If there are no conflicts, then, it might be argued, these features may not be problematic. Furthermore, certain approaches in the field of conflict resolution place emphasis on consensus and resolution and treat consensus as a mark of successful discourse.[4]

However, most conflict practitioners recognize that the absence of overt conflict does not mean an absence of conflict. Nor does it mean an absence of structural problems in the deliberation process. Group discussions and deliberations can be hampered by conflict avoidance or by a range of structural features that prevent participants' concerns from being articulated, explored, validated or assessed for their impact on action strategies. Some of these problematic features relating to professional hierarchy and authority relations have been discussed above. When such discourse structure problems occur, professionals can encounter difficulties in implementing action strategies.

In the field of health care, this problem bears most directly on contexts in which deliberations are held without the direct involvement of patients, clients, their families or advocates. Ethical deliberations among teams of professionals in institutional settings are notable for the absence

---

4. For a discussion of diverse approaches to conflict resolution, see chapter 8.

of participation by patients or clients.[5] If important aspects of the issues have been left unexplored in the discourse, then problems may arise in implementation. Furthermore, if the problems affect people who cannot articulate their response or act on their own behalf, then the problematic aspects of the strategies may go undetected. If difficulties are encountered in implementation, team members whose concerns were not articulated or addressed in the deliberation may hesitate to continue to commit themselves to the agreed-upon course of action. Finally, even when no problems come to light, non-dysfunctional discourse allows practitioners to come to a deeper, more comprehensive, more explicit understanding of when and why their consensus action strategies are good strategies.

It is with this view toward a more comprehensive understanding of the structural elements of discourse that the following discussion of dysfunctional features is proposed. Overall, the most conspicuous structural feature observed in the case conferences concerned the lack of movement through the probing and common-ground stages of the discourse. Conflict researchers have identified a series of stages in discourse in which participants: (1) articulate their diverse positions; (2) probe these positions for underlying interests, concerns, commitments and notions of obligation; (3) explore these underlying concerns for common ground; and (4) formulate action strategies that build on common ground. Practitioners and researchers in this field have observed that conflicts most frequently arise and are exacerbated because of problems in the second and third stages and that discourse which remains on the level of positions and action strategies often fails to get at the root of problems.

In the case deliberations, researchers observed that participants generally articulated varieties of diverse positions, discussed these positions, jumped to action strategies and discussed aspects of implementation. However, in large measure, they skipped the stages involving probing for underlying concerns and the search for common ground, which would

---

5. At various stages of this project, public presentations of interim results elicited the criticism that such ethical deliberations among professionals, in contexts that excluded patients or clients, were inappropriate. The argument in this criticism is that patients/clients must always have a voice in ethical deliberations. What became clear during this project was that, given this argument, there still remains a role for deliberation sessions among professionals in contexts where technical, legal and institutional aspects of issues can be treated quickly in technical language. These sessions can never be the only loci of ethical deliberation. However, they can play an important role in complex ethical deliberations, particularly when discourse is open and constructive and when a variety of professional types bring a wealth of ethically relevant data on diverse aspects of patients'/clients' lives into the deliberations.

support and substantiate their action strategies. In a case where participants did devote considerable discussion to the action strategy, the agreement on action emerged first and was not significantly affected by subsequent probing.

In cases where some probing did occur, the discussions were generally marked by the absence of discourse skills of active listening. Conflict researchers have observed that in the probing and common-ground stages, participants need to listen actively to the words and expressed feelings of each other in order to facilitate the articulation of implicit or felt concerns and values that may be driving the discourse. Furthermore, active listening skills like clarifying, reflecting, restating and validating have the effect of showing the speaker that others have understood and recognized the significance of expressed concerns. This plays an important role in the search for common ground where participants need to be convinced that their concerns have been considered, respected by others and integrated in the aims and objectives for action.

While displays of emotion were frequently visible in the case conferences, participants seldom reflected, validated or probed expressed feelings for their underlying reasons or concerns. In some cases, the expression of emotion was followed by another professional changing the focus of the discussion. Researchers observed few explicit attempts to restate or probe the meaning of statements of others. In some instances, participants interrupted others. Even when these interruptions served to affirm agreement, the effect was to prevent the speaker from exploring significant concerns.

Researchers observed instances of cross talk where participants spoke at each other but spoke past each other. In cross talk, each speaker does not consider and take up the expressed meaning of the previous speaker. In instances where evidence of raised voices and finger pointing suggested overt conflict, no efforts were made to probe the roots of differences. Generally, conversation remained on the level of positions and action strategies.

The goal of this analysis of dysfunctional features is not to criticize the quality of respect showed by the participants toward each other. Rather, conflict research can guide professionals toward understanding and attending to problematic features of discourse even when these features do not result in overt conflict. In health care settings, this can prove most helpful when the routine constraints of professional practice exert a pressure toward efficiency, consensus and action, a pressure that tends to inhibit the exploration of deeper levels of value, which initially may only be apprehended in feelings.

Conflict research provides analytical and practical tools for raising implicit and felt concerns to the level of explicit critical analysis. Clinical deliberations increasingly need to come to grips with complex, multiple value-aspects of health care situations. When professionals encounter these value-aspects in their work, they often experience them first on the level of feelings, notions or hunches that elude explicit articulation. Discourse structure research that pinpoints when such value-aspects are operative implicitly in discourse can help practitioners in the task of ethical analysis. In addition, conflict research prescribes tools, skills and strategies that can help bring such implicit concerns into the arena of explicit, responsible analysis.

ETHICAL STRUCTURE

As was outlined in part 2 of the research, the approach to ethics taken in this project is rooted in the cognitional theory of Bernard Lonergan. To be sure, there is a wide range of theoretical and methodological approaches to ethics in the literature. In the main, the work of Lonergan was chosen because of its potential for integrating the concerns of the two principal schools of thought in discourse ethics, the proceduralists and the contextualists. Lonergan's work identifies four levels of ethical meaning in the overall structure of ethical deliberation. The levels of ethical meaning correspond to the four levels of cognitional operations involved in the apprehension, understanding, judgment and decision of value. Whether the research attends to the procedures of ethical discourse or to the contexts of value implicated in the discourse, this approach finds the fourfold structure relevant to understanding the issues in the cases, the structural dynamics of the deliberation process itself, the activities of participants in the discourse and the operations of the researcher who studies these activities.

In analyzing the case conference videos with the analytical grid of questions constructed from Lonergan's ethical theory, researchers observed evidence of the four levels of ethical meaning. In addition, there seemed to be some correlation between these levels and the four stages of discourse identified by the conflict research. Researchers observed greatest attention to individual desires or positions of the first level of moral meaning and the concrete action strategies that are typical of the fourth level of moral meaning. They found much less attention to the deeper collective or social values and judgments that are found on the second and third levels of moral meaning. First-level values express individual positions and interests and fourth-level values express group action strategies. However, these overt values have their justification in the deeper, more implicit social values of levels two and three. Behind the first- and fourth-level positions and action strategies lie second-level values—the underlying goals and obligations that are rooted in schemes and relations of social order such as professional obligations, institutional roles and responsibilities, legal requirements or family, cultural or religious commitments.[6] Third-level common-good values begin to emerge when each professional begins to articulate their underlying concerns and when the deliberation process allows these concerns to be weighed in relation to each other and subjected to common scrutiny. When the team makes a collective judgment affirming fundamentals of common ground and common direction (third-level value), these fundamentals can set a framework for integrating the various concerns into a framework for action and marshalling reasons justifying some action strategies over others.

When they did appear, second- and third-level values emerged when participants moved through the probing and common-ground stages of discourse structure. First- and fourth-level values (the concrete positions and action strategies held by individuals) tended to arise in the first and fourth stages of discourse structure. In most cases, the participants moved directly from first-level values to fourth-level values, from individual positions to action strategies. However, there was evidence in one case of participants moving more systematically through the various stages of value. Given that this case conference was held after the team had had a chance to read the *Guide for Ethical Deliberation*, the participants may have tried to explicitly follow the recommendations of the guide in this case.

Researchers observed evidence of participants articulating a diverse range of individual positions early on in the case conference and then explicitly probing for some deeper underlying second-level values. At one point, one professional took the opportunity to summarize a range of social, medical, cultural and institutional factors (second-level values) that had been articulated, and to formulate a preliminary common-ground objective (level three) for their program of care. At this point, others intervened to point out expressed concerns that had been overlooked in the summary, to recommend alternative objectives and to assess these objectives in the light of the expressed concerns. Action strategies were evaluated in the light of these common objectives and the discourse came to a close with a sense that all participants would have their concerns met as the strategy was implemented. What was interesting about this particular

---

6.   As was indicated in the discussion of implicit ethics of professions above, participants' concern for professional obligations, institutional roles and responsibilities, and legal requirements were expressed in the videos but they were generally communicated implicitly in statements about details of the cases. In fact, the efforts of researchers to explicate the professional ethics of the various types in the videos in part 1 of this project usually involved the articulation of second-level values in the case conferences.

case conference was that the proposed action strategy involved a team member testing out the proposed program of care with the parents of the child to see if their concerns would be met.

As was noted in the "Implicit Ethics of Professionals" section, above, most of the discourse in this case (and in all the cases) did not involve explicitly ethical language. The various value-aspects of the case tended to be discussed not as instances of wider, recurring ethical relations, but as situation-specific issues that were important because of their bearing on this particular case. However, when the team members began probing for reasons behind the stated positions and weighing the import of various consequences for their proposed programs of care, their deliberations began taking up the tasks of ethics. When participants began asking about the relations among the various values and obligations in the case, they ceased taking for granted any single aspect of the case as normative for action and shifted their concern to determining how the various values could be reconciled in a common strategy.

CONCLUSION

Ethical deliberation brings to light the various value-aspects of issues and seeks to identify how they interrelate and how they bear upon obligations and outcomes. While other forms of discourse implicitly appeal to value notions and terms, ethical discourse focusses attention on these notions and terms and asks whether the assumed values are warranted or grounded. In ordinary discourse or in other forms of technical discourse, value notions tend to be taken for granted. Often, these value notions highlight some parts of the issues and not others. Typically, some aspects of issues are tacitly given priority over others because of the hidden value notions at play in the discourse. However, when participants are not attending to this implicit valuing and prioritizing, important value-aspects of issues can get lost and the significance of more complex and more fundamental values can be inadvertently depreciated.

The task of ethical deliberation is to collectively attend to all of the various value-aspects of cases, to highlight, clarify and reflect on these diverse aspects so that important aspects of human well-being do not get overlooked or violated in formulating action strategies. Ethical analysis aims at formulating and evaluating directions for action that integrate, reconcile and/or prioritize these various value-aspects according to chosen and accepted methods and principles. This can be done implicitly, in the various common-sense or descriptive languages of professions or fields, or it can be done openly and deliberately with the more theoretical concepts, tools and skills of ethics.[7]

The shift to the task of ethics seems to occur when participants begin explicitly probing beyond the various positions for the underlying social values and the grounds for deliberation that will guide the selection and assessment of action strategies. When a variety of professions and types are present in the discourse, this variety tends to be more diverse. When the discourse allows participants to probe, validate and explore the implications of these underlying concerns, questions begin to arise as to how they will be integrated, reconciled or prioritized in a common action strategy. Consequently, it would seem that discourse that encourages and nurtures this exploration of implicit professional values will further the ethical task.

These observations highlight the difference between clinical discourse and ethical discourse. In addition, they help to explain an interesting anomaly or contradictory feature regarding consensus, which arose in the analysis of the case conference videos. As was indicated above, many of the observations in the case conferences were of gestures, forms of professional interaction and features of ethical analysis, which the literature suggests would have a negative impact on the discourse. However, while researchers observed evidence of these dysfunctional features, participants in the case conferences still generally showed little difficulty or hesitation in coming to consensus. Indeed, in many cases, consensus on action strategies emerged early in the discourse. There was a notable lack of overt conflict in the discourse and participants seemed at ease in coming to consensus on action strategies. However, if the research analyses are correct in signalling these various features of the discourse as dysfunctional, then they provide participants with tools for critically evaluating consensus and for asking whether their clinical discourse has adequately dealt with the ethical aspects of the case. Participants need to ask whether the mere fact of consensus is enough or whether the deliberation process has left ethically significant aspects of the case unresolved or unexamined.

Clinical discourse tends to focus on the medical or physiological facts and values of a case. To the extent that health care institutions and legal institutions impose constraints based on wider social values, these other values will also make their way into clinical discourse. When the social atmosphere is litigious, these may even dominate the discourse. However,

---

7. On the relation between common sense and theory, see Bernard Lonergan, *Collected Works of Bernard Lonergan*. vol. 3, *Insight: A Study of Human Understanding*, ed. F. E. Crowe and Robert M. Doran (Toronto: University of Toronto Press, [1957] 1992), 199, 442-445.

ethical discourse opens discussion to the full range of personal, family, institutional, legal, social, cultural, religious and political values of the case, including those that may not be constrained by laws or explicit professional codes. Furthermore, what makes this discourse distinctively ethical is the requirement that no single value-aspect of a case can arbitrarily rule the deliberations.

The call for moving from clinical discourse to ethical discourse may not require introducing hosts of new data into the discussions. The videotaped case conferences of the two health care teams involved in this project revealed evidence of a diverse wealth of positions and value-aspects of the cases that could have been raised to explicit discussion and analysis in the discussions. If these are any indication of the course of typical clinical case conferences, professionals of diverse types can be counted on to introduce adequate data for ethical reflection. It remains for participants in clinical teams to raise this data to explicit analysis and scrutiny in ethical discourse. Even when this ethical analysis does not change the consensus action strategy, it does provide the team with the confidence that the relevant ethical questions have been raised and answered in a satisfactory judgment of the team.

One final point. The literature in ethics abounds with discussions of a variety of methods for integrating, reconciling and/or prioritizing the various and conflicting value-aspects of cases. There would appear to be no emerging consensus on a single approach that would satisfy the concerns of all the major theoretical schools. And, given the current state of the discourse, such a consensus does not seem foreseeable in the near future. This plurality adds a second level of complexity to cases that health care practitioners must deal with. In addition to diverse professional types highlighting diverse value-aspects of cases, they will also highlight diverse theories and methods for treating these diverse and conflicting values. This project has included some discussion of this methodological plurality. However, a word on its import is relevant here.

This study, guided as it is by the theoretical work of Bernard Lonergan, places priority focus on the intelligence and responsibility of women and men who wrestle with the diverse value-aspects of cases in health care teams. Insofar as their group discussions reveal tendencies toward diverse methods of ethical analysis, these methods themselves will tend to highlight diverse value-aspects of the cases that the discussions will need to grapple with. Further research will need to focus on how these diverse methods are revealed in discourse and how practitioners can judge which may be appropriate and when. However, the present analysis is offered as a first step toward this task and as a context within which this task can go forward.

The focus of this project is on moving from implicit to explicit ethics. The goal is to help practitioners become aware of when they are using ethical language, the structure of this language, how this ethical language is embedded in their implicit notions of professional responsibilities, how these implicit normative notions arise in clinical discourse and how an understanding of the structure of discourse can enhance efforts to grapple with them. If this analysis proves helpful, it may suggest a framework for further analysis of ethical methods.

Chapter 10

Guide for Ethical Deliberation

Peter Monette, Kenneth R. Melchin, Tim Flaherty,
Jean-Marc Larouche and Hubert Doucet

The *Guide for Ethical Deliberation* recognizes that the majority of
ethical decisions made in health care settings are the result of deliberations among diverse professionals in health care teams. While hospital
ethics committees are often conspicuously identified with ethical issues,
the full range of issues involved in patient care involves a wide range of
ethical issues that usually remain implicit and are either dealt with or left
unexamined in the deliberations among professionals involved in patient
care. Frequently, members of health care teams encounter difficulties in
talking through concrete ethical issues involving patient care. Just as often, deliberations proceed with the appearance of ease because ethically
significant issues remain unexamined and unresolved. A health care team's
efforts to wrestle with ethical dilemmas sometimes involves overt or cov-
ert conflicts rooted in the dynamics of the deliberation process itself. These
team-rooted conflicts can prove to be difficult obstacles in dealing with
the ethical dimensions of concrete situations.

The *Guide for Ethical Deliberation* is proposed as a tool to help
constructive ethical deliberation in multiprofessional health care teams.
The guide assumes that health care teams will not be aided by outside
ethical consultants or conflict mediators. The guide further assumes that
a health care team's ethical deliberations are informally structured, in
the sense that team members have the liberty to structure the deliberations in whatever way they choose and the authority to implement the
results of the decisions.

The guide was designed in the course of an action-research project
that focussed on ethical issues arising in a pediatric chronic care setting.
However, it is our belief that the usefulness of the guide is not limited to
this context, that it can prove just as helpful to teams of professionals
working in various health care contexts. It is the result of extensive theoretical analysis of implicit ethics in health care professionals, careful study

of ethical theories, an examination of resources from the field of conflict studies and a preliminary "road test" with two teams of health care professionals. The overall framework that integrates these diverse resources is provided by the philosophy of Bernard Lonergan. Yet despite the complexity and diversity of the resources that have been brought together, we have sought to make the guide as user-friendly as possible.

THE NATURE OF ETHICAL DELIBERATION IN HEALTH CARE TEAMS

Technology, public financing and social change are changing the face of health care. Professionals working in health care teams face an increasingly diverse range of ethical issues that often are never explicitly identified as such, yet they shape the course of care. These ethical issues: (1) tend to be increasingly complex involving medical, technological, personal, family, cultural, philosophical, religious, community, institutional, economic and political dimensions; (2) involve a variety of professionals who work in a variety of institutional contexts and who understand their professional obligations toward patient care through the lens of different styles or "types"; (3) often involve a history of encounters and experiences with patients, clients, their families and supporting communities; and (4) often involve conflicts among these multiple ethical aspects.

The result is that deliberation in multiprofessional health care teams needs as much as possible to bring these implicit ethical aspects of cases to the level of explicit awareness, to evaluate their import and to work out a common ground or trajectory for strategies of care. The principal resource for assuring that these ethical concerns are identified and treated responsibly is the diversity of professionals and professional "types" in the team. Each professional has habits of attending to and caring about specific realms of value in the patient's life. Because these habits shape professionals' sense of identity and the direction of their responsibility for care, they focus attention on implicit ethical aspects of patient care that other professionals would not be aware of. This full range of factors must be considered and evaluated in the overall decision making on care. The only way for this to happen is if all professionals participate fully in the deliberation process.

In health care deliberations, no single professional perspective can provide a complete understanding of the ethical issues, cares and concerns. Team members must ensure that the deliberation process will facilitate the articulation of the full range of data, issues and perspectives on the case. Without this full articulation, the team will not be able to meet the demands of the complex ethical problems involved in the case. Quite frequently the only occasion for team members to articulate ethical issues arising within their particular sphere of professional care is in the team's deliberation sessions. Consequently, equal and open dialogue is essential for all members to play their role in ensuring that the full range of issues is dealt with by the team.

The guide assumes that the team members' understanding of the ethical issues in the cases emerge within the dialogue sessions. While all professional perspectives are necessary for common understanding and action, no single perspective is sufficient in itself. Each professional perspective draws on the input of other professions in formatting its own recommendations for care. Consequently, the goal of the dialogue sessions is to integrate the cares and concerns expressed by all team members into a common evaluation of the issues in the case. Only when the dialogue is open and equal can this occur. Thus, the guide assumes that professional relationships among team members contribute toward the common team evaluation.

We have formulated insights into the process and discourse skills that can inform the team's dialogue. We believe that these insights and skills can improve the quality of ethical deliberation. Insights into the process can alleviate the negative effects of power relationships among team members and facilitate open and equal participation. Common action strategies must build upon the common ground that is established in the deliberation process. No member of the team may refrain from or be excluded from articulating the concerns that arise from their professional perspective. Discourse skills can help participants promote effective communication toward mutual understanding on responsible strategies of care.

One final point. A critique often raised against informal or dialogue-based approaches to ethical decision making is that such approaches can never achieve true justice in ethical decisions. The assumption here is that social justice is only the product of fully public dialogue structured by formal or institutional norms and procedures. Critiques of informal dialogue argue that it fails because it is not public and not structured by formally sanctioned norms, regulations, procedures and laws.

Our response to this critique has two parts. First, deliberations and decisions in health care teams are not the only instance of ethical decision making in health care. In fact, the primary locus of ethically relevant discussion and decision is in consultations with patients. In addition, the decisions of health care teams must meet the demands that are articulated within the wider medical-legal environments of hospitals and the related institutions where the various professionals are accountable. Finally, these institutional decisions are themselves accountable to wider sets of legal, academic, social, media and political arenas. All of these in one way or another can and do affect ethical decision making of teams and can act as a corrective to bias in team members. Second, ethical discussions among team members are often the place where a great deal of constructive ethical analysis can take place. When high-quality ethical deliberation takes place within health care teams, important ethical issues can often be dealt with before they become seriously disruptive for patients and institutions. Since various professionals are often sensitive to different dimensions of patient care, open and fair dialogue can often result in these issues being expressed and integrated in strategies of care. The guide is proposed as a means for helping such health care team integration and not as a replacement or subversion of more formal justice processes.

Guide for Ethical Deliberation

Section 1: The Four Levels of Value in Ethical Deliberation

Section 2: The Process of Ethical Deliberation

Section 3: Skills for Ethical Deliberation

Section 4: Self-Assessment Guide

Section 1: The Four Levels of Value in Ethical Deliberation

Introduction

When health care professionals come together to discuss ethical concerns arising in clinical cases, they bring diverse professional concerns to the process, yet they seek a team consensus that is founded upon mutual understanding. Research has shown that the process of ethical deliberation has a structure. Awareness of this structure can be used to help guide team dialogue.

The Four Levels of Value

In ethical deliberation, the focus rests on the types or levels of value that are at stake in the case under discussion. There are four distinct but interrelated levels of value. On the first level of value are the *individual positions*. They are what we want out of the dialogue. On the second level are the underlying cares and concerns that are the foundations of our positional values. We can call these *individual underlying values*. Frequently these values exist on a feeling level and are not articulated by the participants.

In ethical deliberation the values of a single professional are not usually sufficient to deal with the complexities of the issues at hand. These complexities require dialogue among a wide range of professionals. Thus, in deliberation sessions a number of different individual positional values supported by a number of individual underlying values are expressed. The deliberation process needs to aim at integrating these diverse values into a common viewpoint. Through mutual understanding, integration and collective decision, the team can achieve a common set of cares and concerns that represent the team's values. This is the third level of value and we call these *team underlying values*. From these values the team is able to develop new cooperative action strategies. These action strategies are the fourth level of value, and we call them *team action strategies*.

The Four Levels of Value

	Individual Values	Team Values
Positions and Action Strategies	First Level of Value *Individual Positions* Events 1-2. **Phase 1: Articulation**	Fourth Level of Value *Team Action Strategies* Events 6-7. **Phase 4: Implementation**
Underlying Cares and Concerns	Second Level of Value *Individual Underlying Values* Event 3. **Phase 2: Validation**	Third Level of Value *Team Underlying Values* Events 4-5. **Phase 3: Integration**

Section 2: The Process of Ethical Deliberation

Introduction

Ethical dialogue is structured into four phases. Each phase has a goal that the dialogue must achieve in order for the team to adequately move through the structure of dialogue. Each phase is then broken down into events. Events further orientate the teams' dialogue toward more specific goals.

The Four Phases of the Process of Ethical Deliberation

There are four phases to the process of ethical deliberation. They are: *articulation*, *validation*, *integration* and *implementation*.

The *articulation* phase aims to have each participant in the dialogue express his or her position on the case so that all team members can hear their views.

The *validation* phase allows the team to identify and affirm the cares and concerns that arise from each participant's professional involvement in the case. This phase is not concerned with judging whether a participants' position is correct or incorrect. Rather, the aim here is to move beyond the individual positions that were stated in the articulation phase in order to bring out the underlying cares and concerns of each participant. The validation phase aims to show that each participant's place in the dialogue is important and that their views must be considered by all in order for the team to address the complexities of the situation at hand.

The *integration* phase allows all the participants of the dialogue to appreciate and understand each other's cares and concerns. From this mutual understanding there is formulated a collective viewpoint or framework that represents the team's central values on the case. Evaluation of the team's common goals in the case ensures that this team consensus responds to all the individual concerns expressed in the validation phase.

The *implementation* phase aims to allow the team to formulate action strategies that will meet the cares and concerns reflected by all of the professional perspectives of the members of the team.

The Seven Events of the Deliberation Process

To achieve the goals of the four phases, the team must move through *seven events*. They are: (1) opening the dialogue; (2) expressing individual positions; (3) probing for underlying concerns; (4) seeking understanding toward common ground; (5) evaluating the team consensus; (6) brainstorming alternative solutions; and (7) finalizing team action strategies.

In the discussion of events, we begin to see the correlation between the four levels of value and the structure of the deliberation process.

PHASE 1: ARTICULATION

Event 1: *Opening the dialogue* refers simply to the process of allowing the team to discuss rules that allow for equal participation.

Event 2: *Expressing individual positions* aims to allow each participant the opportunity to tell the whole team exactly what his or her position is on the issues.

PHASE 2: VALIDATION

Event 3: *Probing for underlying concerns* allows the team to move beyond the initial positions of each participant to the underlying cares and concerns that form the reasons for one's positions. This event requires that each participant be encouraged to articulate their cares and concerns. In their interaction the team members seek to appreciate and validate each other as participants in search of common understanding and action in response to the demands of the case.

PHASE 3: INTEGRATION

Event 4: *Seeking understanding toward common ground* aims to achieve mutual understanding among all members. From such understanding there is the possibility that there will emerge a collective viewpoint that expresses the team's central values. With this collective viewpoint the dialogue can move to team action.

Event 5: *Evaluating the team consensus* allows the team to decide whether their common framework is indeed a good framework. A framework is good when it addresses all the team members' concerns that are expressed in event 3.

PHASE 4: IMPLEMENTATION

Event 6: *Brainstorming alternative solutions* allows the team to search for the widest range of possible ways of implementing the team consensus. The aim is simply to articulate all possible solutions without judging the validity of any specific solution.

Event 7: *Finalizing team action strategies* aims to allow the team to decide on the action strategy they will implement. The team must select which action strategy will most effectively meet their common cares and concerns that emerged in event 4. Common action strategies should link up what the team wants to achieve with specific responsibilities for all affected participants.

The Process of Ethical Deliberation

Phase 1: Articulation

Event 1. Opening the dialogue
Event 2. Expressing individual positions

Phase 2: Validation

Event 3. Probing for underlying concerns

Phase 3: Integration

Event 4. Seeking understanding toward common ground
Event 5. Evaluating the team consensus

Phase 4: Implementation

Event 6. Brainstorming alternative solutions
Event 7. Finalizing team action strategies

Section 3: Skills for Ethical Deliberation

Introduction

Successful ethical deliberation depends upon the way participants in a team interact. Communication skills play an important role in the deliberation since they both allow the speaker to articulate his or her thoughts and help the listener to accurately understand what the speaker has intended. Communication, however, is not usually a skill that one has deliberately developed and refined. This means that the quality of our dialogue is often less than what we would like it to be. The following two communication skills are helpful for effective mutual understanding. They can be incorporated into all stages of a team's deliberations.

Turn Taking

Turn taking is the basic skill in ethical dialogue. It involves simply two interchanging roles, speaker and listener. The speaker's role is to articulate his or her thoughts in such a way that the listener will be able to understand what the speaker intends to communicate. The listener's role is to actively listen to the speaker's words and intention. Although these two roles are easy enough to understand, they are often difficult to implement in actual dialogue. Oftentimes the intensity of our dialogue prohibits us from allowing the other person to say what he or she wants to say. Sometimes we find ourselves talking at each other rather than seeking to really listen to what the other person is communicating. Therefore, both the speaker and the listener roles require a willingness to engage in the dialogue in such a way that the discourse will move forward toward the team common framework.

Restating

Restating is an active listening technique that can be quite effective in dialogue. It involves the listener telling the speaker what the speaker has just attempted to communicate to the listener. The restating skill is not a normal practice in our daily conversations. Usually, once someone has finished speaking we take this as an opportunity for our turn to talk. Sometimes we respond to the other with the phrase, "Yes, but" and then continue to tell the speaker what we think. However, before we can respond to the speaker, we must check out with the speaker that we understand correctly what the speaker has intended by his or her words. This is not simply telling the speaker that we understand him or her. Rather, it involves restating our understanding in our own words and asking the speaker to confirm if this is, indeed, what he or she meant. The skill of restating is particularly important when an issue is highly conflictual. The conflict signals to the participants that an issue is important for one or more participants. It is the importance of the issue that demands that all participants accurately understand each other. Accurate understanding occurs by allowing each speaker to confirm that he or she has been correctly understood by other participants.

Section 4: Self-Assessment Guide

The following questions allow each participant to foster awareness of his or her participation in ethical dialogue. Answer each question as completely as you can. Only you will see your answers. You can use this assessment guide both before and after your team dialogue.

1. What are your individual positions concerning the case at issue?

2. What are your individual underlying values (reasons, cares and concerns)? How are these related to your sense of your professional goals and responsibilities with regard to the case?

3. How are your individual positions related to your underlying values? How can you articulate these underlying values for the other team members?

4. How have other team members helped you appreciate different aspects of the case? Can you rethink or reformulate your positions and concerns in relation to those expressed by other professionals? Are you prepared to reassess or change your mind on aspects of the case?

5. Which possible points of view are you willing to listen to? Which professionals are the most difficult for you to listen to? Are there individuals or types of individuals that you find difficult to talk with? How do you usually deal with such people? Can you find something in the ideas of these other professionals that you can affirm as important? Can you find action strategies that build upon this common ground?

6. Can you distinguish a participant's individual positional value from the person him- or herself? If so, how?

Chapter 11

Thinking About Ethical Deliberation in Multiprofessional Health Care Teams

Kenneth R. Melchin

The goal of this chapter is to stand back and reflect on the whole project, to ask about the overall framework that guided the research and developed through the project and to examine how this framework unified the various parts of the project. While the theoretical literature in ethics is massive and diverse, three central concerns guided the development of the theoretical framework.

The first concern was linked to the two practical goals of the project: (1) to help understand value conflicts and ethical decision making in the concrete experiences of multiprofessional health care teams; and (2) to develop tools that would assist these teams in their ethical deliberation.

The second concern arose from the first stage of the research. Ethical values are often implicit in the discourse of health care teams. These implicit values often seem to drive the ethical discourse quite apart from the parties' explicit focus on the issues. For the most part, these implicit values are linked to the way the parties understand their professional goals and commitments.

The third concern arose from observations from research and practice in health care teams. Most often, ethical discourse in health care teams involves conflicts. Consequently, we turned to the field of conflict studies for conceptual and practical tools to analyze conflicts and to help practitioners in working with value conflicts.

Given the practical goals of the research, the conflictual nature of the ethical dialogue in this milieu and the concern with the role of implicit ethics in shaping the course of this conflictual discourse, the project needed a theoretical framework that could guide the research in an orderly way and facilitate integrating these diverse concerns into a single, comprehensive viewpoint.

Diverse Streams in Ethical Theory

Chapter 6, by James Sauer, in this volume presents a brief overview and analysis of some of the principal contributors to the theoretical literature in ethics. Scholars have identified two main currents in this literature, which Sauer calls the contextualists and the proceduralists.

The focus of the contextualists (e.g., Gadamer, MacIntyre, Sandel) is on the social, cultural, historical traditions and contexts of meaning that inform ethical claims and that set the framework for adjudicating among conflicting claims (e.g., cultures, religious traditions, professions, ethical theories, social movements, institutions, structures of practice). Foundational norms or principles for resolving ethical disputes are not to be found in the analysis of universal, formal structures but in the analysis of spheres and cultural contexts of ethical meaning, which the parties implicitly draw upon in advancing their claims. The contextualists argue that purely formal or discourse-structure approaches themselves draw upon traditions for their notions of obligation and rationality and that a full grounding of their own theories requires appropriating these traditions.

The focus of the proceduralists (e.g., Habermas, Rawls, Ackerman) is on the structures and institutions of ethical discourse. Their interest is in general structural features, which operate in all ethical discourse regardless of context or ethical content. The analysis of these structural features seeks to identify general norms or obligations, which are rooted in the discourse structure itself. All participants are rationally bound to accept these norms or obligations whenever they seek to advance their ethical claims through discourse.

Sauer's chapter draws upon the work of Paul Ricoeur to argue that these two theoretical currents do not present mutually exclusive analyses of ethical discourse. Rather, they highlight two realms of normativity that are operative in ethical discourse and that interact to drive the dynamics of discourse in complex dialectical ways. To understand what is going on in discourse requires analyzing both the interpersonal contexts of moral meaning (usually implicitly) operative in the discourse and the more general procedural dynamics of the discourse process.

Sauer's analysis does not put an end to the hosts of theoretical debates in ethics. However, his analysis does provide a fertile heuristic to guide research. If these two theoretical currents do not offer conflicting analyses of the same phenomena but complementary analyses of distinct realms of norms operative in ethical deliberation, then research would need to analyze discourse in both realms. These two realms would need to be reflected in formulating practical guides for ethical deliberation.

The research of part 1 of the project, the results of which are presented in the chapters by Jean-Marc Larouche and Tim Flaherty, represents a contextualist approach to ethical discourse. The normativity of the ethical claims of the various professionals is grounded in the specific context of meaning operative in the implicit self-understanding of each professional type. Furthermore, the dynamic interactions among the various professionals arise not only from general features of discourse itself but also from the specific conflicts and complementarities among the meaning contexts of the professional types. For health care teams to deal effectively with ethical conflicts, professionals must understand the implicit ethical claims of their own professional types and recognize the same in others. Furthermore, in situations of conflict, they need to move beyond the limitations of these contexts and strive to find common ethical horizons. The contextualist analysis would suggest that such common horizons are to found in an understanding of the wider social and institutional contexts, which set the common environment for their professional interaction.

Chapter 8, by Peter Monette, in part 2 of this volume, summarizes research in the field of conflict studies and represents a proceduralist approach to ethical discourse. Conflict analysts and practitioners are not concerned principally with the cultural or professional contexts of meaning of the value claims of the parties in the discourse. Rather, their concern is to identify and rectify structural dysfunctions in the discourse process that exacerbate conflicts and present barriers to the exploration of common horizons of meaning and value. The analysis of the stages of conflictual discourse yields common procedural norms for guiding the parties through the stages of the deliberation process. The analysis of discourse skills yields tools that can help the parties through this process.

While Sauer's analysis suggests a complementarity between these two lines of research, the question remains as to how these two realms of normativity come together in concrete, ethical deliberation. Ethical deliberation in health care teams needs to result in an outcome, an action strategy, an agreement that brings the discourse to closure. If the two lines of analysis yield two realms of normativity operative in discourse, then theorists and practitioners need to understand how these two realms function together in ethical deliberation to yield single outcomes. This research project looked to the philosophy of Bernard Lonergan for an overarching theoretical framework for unifying the diverse aspects of the research and for understanding the interactions among the diverse realms of normativity in ethical deliberation.

THE ETHICAL THEORY FRAMEWORK OF
BERNARD LONERGAN

Lonergan's philosophy is based upon four distinct levels of operations that seem to be involved in human cognition. While Lonergan developed his fourfold structure in the study of cognition as operative in scientific understanding, his own work and that of others has carried this forward into a theory of ethics.

Lonergan describes the four levels as experience, understanding, judgment and decision. In any type of inquiry, the first level is experience, which presents ideas, hunches, problems to be solved, data to be examined and feelings to be explored. The move to the second level, to the operations of understanding, takes the materials of experience and views them in a new light. In the effort to understand things, we stop taking them for granted and start examining them, probing them, looking for an underlying unity to the data, an intelligibility that links the parts together into a whole. The driving force of understanding is questions and the product is insights. However, insights often yield only partial, incomplete or even misleading aspects of things. Consequently, the third level involves judgment, the critical scrutiny of our insights in search of linkages and a more comprehensive understanding that satisfies the demands of our inquiring. Here, we want to know if the insights stand the test of our questions and experiences. When we find holes in our insights, when we find them partial, when we find them problematic, we go back to experience in search of clues for new insights. When judgment proclaims the full set of insights to stand up to our collective questioning, we move on to decision and action. The fourth level involves putting things into practice.

When the inquiry is ethical, the distinctions among the four levels of operations mean that the term "value" takes on different meanings as we move from one level to another. On the first level, the level of interest or desire, the good is the object of our immediate, practical desire. In team deliberations, discourse on this level yields diverse interests, objectives and positions. Here is where ethical diversity and conflict first appear.

On the second level of social order, ethical language comes to mean something different. Here, we cease taking the immediate practical desires and objectives for granted as the last word. We begin questioning, probing, looking for reasons. Our search is for reasons why we want what we want and we find answers through understanding social relations. Ethical language on this second level refers to the social orders, institutions and relations that ground our desires and obligations and justify what we want.

The third level arises when we discover that ethical understanding can be partial, be multiple and yield diverse and conflicting answers to questions. At this point our concerns shift to the task of evaluation and judgment. Because most ethical discourse involves multiple parties, the task at this level is to find a common perspective for integrating or reconciling the various understandings of the various parties. Here we seek to identify the wider goals of justice or well-being that express directions of progress for society at large. Furthermore, ethical evaluation requires assessing proposed solutions to see if they respond to all of the requirements of social, historical justice, even when these may not be articulated in legal or professional codes. This can be the most difficult level of ethical deliberation, the level on which the most theoretical diversity arises. However, if the parties in the discourse bring a sufficiently diverse range of concerns to the table, and if the discourse is open and constructive, parties will find resources for evaluation in the range of social or professional values expressed in the discourse.[1]

The fourth level of value involves commitment, decision and action. Here, ethical language refers to the practical action strategies that are formulated to implement the results of the deliberations. Decision requires more than an affirmation of value, it requires a commitment to action at specific times with specific divisions of labour. Decisions may be agreed to informally, but they may also be articulated in formal contracts and agreements that are mutually recognized as binding. In either case, what distinguishes this level of value are its specific obligations for action.

The cognitional theory of Lonergan suggests a framework for understanding the points of contact between the contextualist and proceduralist lines of analysis of ethical discourse. If Lonergan is correct, both approaches will reveal participants in discourse implementing the various levels of cognitional operations at different moments. Clearly, the two lines of analysis will reveal different aspects and features of ethical deliberation. However, Lonergan's framework suggests that a search for points of contact could yield insights for integrating the contributions of both.

---

1. In Lonergan's cognitional theory, judgment involves raising and answering the range of relevant questions. Furthermore, judgments about what is relevant and what constitutes appropriate answers to such questions will sometimes challenge the integrity and personal value stances of the interlocutors. Invariably, pediatric chronic care cases will raise questions about oppression and victimization of powerless individuals and minorities. These questions and concerns are a legitimate part of ethical deliberations. However, whether they are to be accorded dominant or minor priority in the evaluation is not decided *a priori*. It is only decided in the deliberations through the dedicated deliberations of people. See Bernard Lonergan, *Method in Theology* (New York: Herder and Herder, 1973), chaps. 1, 10 and 11.

In this study, the teams worked relatively independently through the first stage of the research and then came together more directly during the second. It was during the second case conference analysis stage that researchers began reflecting on the points of contact between their diverse approaches. The following discussion offers a set of insights into these points of contact. This discussion is not meant to be exhaustive. Rather, it seeks to initiate a line of discussion that promises to contribute to both theory and practice in ethics. The goal is to provide clues on when and where diverse lines of analysis are engaged in a common enterprise. If Lonergan's insights can help clarify the shape and texture of ethical deliberation in its various stages, then it will yield tools for bringing the fruits of diverse theoretical approaches to bear upon a common project.

Finally, this discussion does not offer a simplistic formula for resolving complex theoretical and practical disputes in pediatric chronic care. The foundation for ethical judgment and decision in the work of Bernard Lonergan is the responsibility and authenticity of the women and men who wrestle with the concrete complexities of ethical issues. As in the common-law legal tradition, the product of these ongoing judgments is an accumulating body of insights and judgments that are found to stand the test of time. Lonergan's approach precludes any type of analysis that would bypass this process of concrete deliberation. What it does offer is some clarity of understanding on what participants in ethical deliberation are doing at each stage in a discourse. It is toward this goal of clarity that the following discussions are offered.

POINTS OF CONTACT BETWEEN THE DIVERSE STREAMS IN ETHICAL THEORY

A number of points of contact between the proceduralist (conflict analysis) and contextualist (implicit ethics of professions) lines of research were observed.

First, while the two analyses have different points of focus, they both seek to distinguish explicit from implicit ethics. Both look beyond the foreground of personal ethical positions and claims to the implicit background of social or discourse relations whose analysis would yield criteria for reconciling conflicting claims. Furthermore, while both focus on this distinction between explicit and implicit ethics, both locate the principal forces driving disputes and the resources for resolution in the realm of the implicit. For both, it is the implicit which is the most significant. It is the implicit which tends to drive the discourse, often quite apart from the participants' explicit positions or claims. And it is the analysis of the implicit which provides the wider framework for understanding and adjudicating claims.

This concern with implicit normativity, whether it arises from professional contexts or from the structure of the discourse itself, suggests a distinction between levels of value that would seem to correspond to Lonergan's insights into the levels of cognition in ethics. The terms "ethical" and "value" have distinct levels of meaning. The first pertains to the concrete, practical objectives that the parties seek to attain. This is the level of value as *interest*. The second pertains to a deeper, more complex structure of meanings or relations that set the backdrop or the environment for these objectives. This is the level of value as *social order*. Both proceduralists and contextualists argue that ethical disputes cannot be settled on the first level of value. It is only in probing the second level that self-understanding is deepened, mutual understanding is sought and conflicting claims can be reconciled rationally.

Second, despite their differences, both lines of analysis highlight the *social character of value* on the second level of moral meaning, which comes to light in the analysis of implicit ethics. Both find the deeper context of normativity to lie in a shared sociality whose structures are structures of shared meaning and whose internal coherence or dynamic logic sets the framework for evaluating claims on the first level of value.

To be sure, the social structures of the conflict and professional-type analyses are different. Conflict discourse structures are dynamic structures of interpersonal or institutional interaction whose fundamental logic is the dynamic scheme of conversation itself. The social structures of the various professional types, on the other hand, seem to be concrete meaning structures of a different sort. They seem to be social ecologies of meaning in which professionals make commitments to clients, to other professionals, to administrators and to the public at large. These commitments find their rationale in specific sets of social routines constituted by extant technologies, health care institutions, cultural expectations and institutions of politics and law.

However, what is interesting is that for both lines of analysis, the wider, deeper context of normativity that will illuminate and evaluate concrete value claims will be revealed in probing the social meaning structures that set the playing field on which individuals make their claims.

Third, in both lines of analysis there is an important role for detecting and exploring *feelings* in moving from the first, explicit level to the second, implicit level of value. In both cases, implicit values are not articulated directly, but tend to be revealed indirectly, either in literature or in discourse, through rhetorical technique, emotionally charged language, innuendo or body language, all of which express feelings. It is the exploration of these expressed feelings which leads the analyst from explicit to implicit ethics. Furthermore, the supposition of both lines of analysis is that the feelings reveal values that shape the behaviour of the parties even though they may not be articulated or even understood by the parties themselves.

The implication here is that the transition from the first to the second level of ethical analysis involves not only understanding social meaning structures in a purely abstract sense but also self-discovery in an existential sense. Both lines of analysis seem to presuppose that feelings reveal values embedded in the structures of our actual social living that shape our living but may often be at odds with our explicit valuing. If ethical analysis is the total social activity in which we articulate to ourselves our implicit social valuing, then exploring implicit values revealed through feelings will be self-discovery. It will be discovery not only of things we ought to value, but things we actually do value in the routines of our daily living. It is bringing this valuing to light through the analysis of feeling, subjecting it to careful scrutiny and testing its coherence with our valuing in other dimensions of our own lives and the lives of others which seems to be the goal of both proceduralist and contextualist lines of ethical analysis.

Fourth, both lines of ethical analysis seem to presuppose a difference between the analytic attitude of exploring, understanding, explaining values and the normative attitude of scrutinizing, evaluating, adjudicating and judging these values. The form of this second, evaluative activity is different in the proceduralist and contextualist lines of analysis. But both presuppose a difference in attitudes. This common presupposition suggests a third level of meaning to ethical language, a level that moves beyond the second analytic level to the critical goal of *evaluation and judgment*. This corresponds to Lonergan's third level of cognition in ethics.

In both cases, the criteria for the reflective activity of scrutinizing and judging seems to be some form of rational and existential coherence between our explicit value claims and the wider social ecology of value that is revealed in our collective implicit ethics. To be sure, achieving this coherence is far more than simply a matter of logical analysis. Nor are the roads to this goal understood similarly by the two lines of analysis. For the proceduralist, coherence involves the parties recognizing and decisively accepting the obligations of implicit performative or linguistic claims, which we make on each other whenever we engage in discourse in civil society or whenever we draw upon the fruits of a society built upon this discourse. For the contextualist, coherence involves the parties recognizing and decisively accepting the obligations implicit in the ecologies of meaning, which set the institutions of our living and which are the bedrock on which we stand when we make our individual value claims. However, what is similar is the requirement of coherence itself.

What is interesting about this notion of coherence is that in neither approach is the implied coherence simply a conformity of self to other or vice versa. Rather, the implied coherence seems to be between two dimensions of our own living, our *explicit* value claims and the *implicit* obligations of our lived sociality. Because this living is social, coherence with the implied structures of sociality grounds the possibility of our living with others. Consequently, the higher level of value is the social.[2] Furthermore, when values implicit in our wider social living are revealed to conflict with those of other groups, the task of evaluation and judgment must look to wider and deeper structures of lived social order for evaluative criteria.

Fifth, a common supposition of both approaches is that the conflicting parties and groups will find evaluative criteria for reconciling or adjudicating conflicting value claims by articulating a *common good*. Again, the realm where this common good is sought differs in the two approaches. But their concern for common ground is shared. When implicit values of diverse cultural or professional contexts are found to conflict dramatically, then finding common notion of the good may require exploring quite new forms of communal or institutional living. Consequently the common good may not always be already-lived common ground. However, the common good is never totally new. It always has its roots in lived values, which are embedded in past and present structures of social living. And it is to these actual lived contexts that the parties appeal when they specify requirements that the new order must meet.

The proceduralist tends to rely on extant analyses of discourse structures for their evaluative criteria for common ground. However, even when they do, the structural demands of the deliberation process may force considerable creativity and innovation in articulating common ground. Here, I would argue, the two lines of analysis most clearly need each other. The most immediate, palpable common ground for conflicting parties is to be found in the actual discourse itself. If parties are to avoid violence and to choose discourse to settle major value conflicts, then their most immediate common good is their mutual commitment to the deliberation process. However, if this process is to go forward constructively, the parties will need the most comprehensive and creative analyses of the contexts of social meaning implicated in the cases or issues

---

2. This does not imply sacrificing individuals to society. On the contrary, democratic forms of sociality require a respect for persons as integral to the dynamics of social routines. Theories based on rights place generalized rights over merely particular claims of individuals that would infringe on these rights. This is a claim to the priority of social value over individual values. For a discussion of this priority see, Kenneth R. Melchin, *Living with Other People: An Introduction to Christian Ethics Based on Bernard Lonergan* (Ottawa: Novalis; Collegeville: Liturgical Press, 1998).

to find common grounds for living out their diverse concerns. And, to be sure, the commitment to discourse must find a fundamental place within the horizons of meaning of the parties.

What seems to be suggested here is that a vision of the common good sets the framework for working out the third level of value. This common good must be both procedural and contextual. When it is procedural, it is the common commitment to the obligations of the discourse which specifies the requirements that all parties must meet. While this common commitment may say little about the actual issues that are the focus of the parties' explicit concern, it does establish the process of working out value differences toward common action strategies.

When the common good is understood contextually, the parties accept the obligation to respect the central values that each articulates in their diverse professional contexts of meaning. But they also accept the obligation to find a common social terrain in which these diverse values can be lived together. This may mean returning to a common heritage. But it may also mean innovation when the common terrain for reconciling these diverse values is not to be found in the past or present. In this case, the commitment to common ground means a commitment to search collectively for forms of collective living that live up to and respect these demands. While the particular value demands of individuals and groups may undergo some modification in the process of working out common ground, it is the demand of equity rooted in the proceduralist's discourse criteria that keeps this modification from capitulating to the constraints of power.

Sixth, the final point of contact between the proceduralist and contextualist streams of analysis involves the turn to implementation, commitment, action, signing agreements, parcelling out tasks, setting the project in motion and calling for everyone's commitment to carry out their designated tasks. This concern for action, for implementation, is a different kind of commitment than those found in the earlier stages of ethical deliberation. Where the second level of value implied a commitment to understanding implicit values, and where the third level called for a commitment to judging or adjudicating conflicting claims in the light of common ground, this is a fourth level of value, which calls for a *commitment to action.* Here, the tasks involve brainstorming, finalizing action strategies and deciding which courses of action best realize the formulated objectives of the team. This corresponds to Lonergan's fourth level of cognition in ethics, the level of decision and action.

What is interesting is that this final stage results in concrete action strategies, which, in some cases, may not look significantly different from the concrete practical objectives that were the explicit object of individual parties in the first stages of the discourse described above. However, what is different about this final stage is that now the practical action is mutual, it reflects the team's objectives and not simply those of one individual. Furthermore, now the action strategies are the product of analysis and deliberation, which has probed the underlying social ecologies within which these strategies find their rationale. Consequently, if all has gone well to this point, team members can give themselves over to implementation and action with a new resolve.

THE GUIDE FOR ETHICAL DELIBERATION

The *Guide for Ethical Deliberation* was constructed on the basis of four theoretical suppositions drawn from the fields of research that were brought together in the ethical theory framework of this project. Clearly, these theoretical suppositions reflect the points of contact discussed above and they reveal the influence of the philosophy of Bernard Lonergan. Members of the research team were able to find anecdotal evidence to support their relevance in the case conference videos of the health care teams. Furthermore, as these discussions show, they were able to discern lines of correlation in the three lines of research that would seem to add additional support to these suppositions.

The first of these suppositions concerns the relevance of *implicit values of diverse professional types*. The guide was constructed on the theoretical supposition that much ethical deliberation is shaped by the participants' implicit understanding of their own professional commitments and obligations. In case conference deliberations these implicit obligations and commitments tend to focus a professional's attention toward data and values that are related to his or her own type. The guide is dedicated to helping health care professionals raise their implicit professional values to the level of explicit reflection in their case conference deliberations. To this end, some tools are presented in section 4 of the guide, in the "Self-Assessment Guide." And further research would most certainly reveal a more detailed set of tools that could aid professionals in health care teams (see "Recommendations for Further Research" below).

Apart from the few tools mentioned above, there is little direct reference to this first supposition in the *Guide for Ethical Deliberation*. However, the import of this supposition is woven into every aspect of the guide. The guide is constructed on the assumption that the clarification of implicit professional commitments and obligations will reveal to all members of the team diverse value-aspects of a case that could well remain hidden from professionals individually. When professionals weigh and prioritize diverse value-aspects of cases, they do so in large measure on the basis of their own personal sense of professional obligations. These, of necessity, are often quite limited. To ensure that discourse brings to light and legitimates all ethically relevant data, the team needs to ensure that all perspectives are heard and recognized openly and equally.

The second theoretical supposition, whose import is ever-present throughout the guide, concerns the *structure of ethical deliberation process*. Researchers, drawing from the field of conflict resolution, have identified four general stages in the structure of discourse. Each stage involves operations that are essential to constructive ethical deliberation. Each stage has a distinctive goal and participants can focus their discussions toward common objectives by identifying where they are at any point in the discourse and attending to the relevant goal. Since the stages need to unfold cumulatively and progressively, each set of operations building upon the fruits of the previous stage, participants can be cautious of moving too quickly through essential stages or of skipping stages. Finally, the stage analysis can provide participants with tools toward diagnosing the roots of problems when discourse encounters difficulties or breaks down.

In the guide, these four stages are presented as the four phases of ethical deliberation: articulation, validation, integration and implementation. To help practitioners implement these insights, these four phases are further broken down into seven events. Phase 1, articulation, involves: (1) opening the dialogue and (2) expressing individual positions. Phase 2, validation, involves: (3) probing for underlying concerns. Phase 3, integration, involves: (4) seeking understanding toward common ground and (5) evaluating the team consensus. And phase 4, implementation, involves: (6) brainstorming alternative solutions and (7) finalizing team action strategies.

The third theoretical supposition concerns the relevance of discourse skills, which are drawn from the field of conflict resolution. Two of these skills, turn taking and restating, are introduced in section 3 of the guide. Clearly, many more could be discussed. While these may initially seem simplistic, the supposition is that skills can help participants to attend explicitly to the discourse of others, to restate the meanings of others, to clarify misunderstandings and to reflect to others that their meanings have been understood correctly and appreciated. When this happens, discourse tends to unfold more in a pattern of real dialogue where participants learn from each other, where the discourse builds relationships and where the end product is an enrichment and development of each individual's original position. Authentic ethical dialogue is a collaborative effort and the supposition here is that discourse skills enhance the quality of this collaboration by allowing each person's ethical deliberations to benefit from those of others.

The fourth theoretical supposition pertains most directly to the cognitional theory of Bernard Lonergan. The supposition here is that ethics is not confined to feelings; is not a logical process of deducing from first principles; is not a purely personal matter, nor purely procedural or entirely contextual; is not totally reducible to power and domination; and is not arbitrary contracting. Rather, ethics consists in women and men bringing a set of cognitional operations to bear upon concrete issues and subjecting first-level value notions and feelings to a set of transformations and clarifications in a structure of collaborative discourse.

The supposition from the philosophy of Lonergan is that ethical operations unfold on four levels, and in ethical deliberation participants must move collectively through these four levels of operations to transform ethical notions into ethical knowledge, judgments and decisions. The goals of these four sets of operations have been found to correspond, roughly, to the four stages of discourse from the field of conflict resolution. Discourse skills aid participants in moving through this collective effort. Throughout the deliberation process the patterns of caring and valuing that arise from implicit professional types need to be articulated and recognized by all as important contributions to ethical reflection but as partial insights that need to be integrated into a common perspective. The elaboration of this common perspective is the goal of ethical deliberation.

In the *Guide for Ethical Deliberation*, these four levels of cognitional operations are identified as levels of value and are referred to as "individual positions," "individual underlying values," "team underlying values" and "team action strategies." The shift that Lonergan calls a shift from insight to judgment arises most frequently in ethical discourse in the effort to reconcile and adjudicate diverse and conflicting concerns of individuals. The transition from insight to judgment seems to occur most often in the transition from multiple concerns articulated by individuals to a common framework elaborated and evaluated by the group.

RECOMMENDATIONS FOR FURTHER RESEARCH

Clearly the goals and achievements of this research have been limited. Given the complexity of the issues in health care, given the diversity of lines of research that have been brought together in this project, given the efforts to bring together practical and theoretical goals and given the novelty of the approach, the research can offer only preliminary conclusions and point toward further lines of inquiry and verification. The following recommendations are based on both a critical assessment of the limits of this project and a confidence in lines of further research that would advance its aims.

(1) The first and most obvious recommendation is linked to the methodological limits of this project. Further research would need to subject the preliminary and anecdotal observations of this project to empirically rigorous testing to verify the relevance of the three lines of literature research to case conference ethical discourse in health care teams. Because of the limits of this project, these researchers neither intended nor were they able to carry out empirically controlled quantitative research.

However, the results of this project would suggest that this next stage is both possible and warranted. There seems to be a linkage between the implicit ethical types of professionals and their habits of attention and values prioritization in ethical discourse. Furthermore, there seems to be a correlation between the dynamic structure and relevant skills of conflicts and ethical discourse. Finally, the fourfold cognitional structure from the work of Lonergan would seem to offer a theoretical framework for this research. These provisional conclusions can be and need to be subjected to empirical verification using the quantitative methods of the social sciences.

(2) The second recommendation, which would seem to be the most relevant to the concrete practice of practitioners in pediatric chronic care, concerns the relevance of the theoretical observations in this research to the concrete issues in this field. While the preparation of the case studies involved detailed research into the concrete ethical issues of this field, the analysis of the project did not include concrete insights on the issues in the case conference deliberations.

This research, based as it is on Lonergan's cognitional theory, does not assume that all ethical judgments will result in a harmonious coordination of conflicting values. However, this project has not offered practitioners tools for differentiating between situations that admit such a coordination and others that require a ranking of values or even a rejection of false value-aspects of cases. This line of further research is essential.

What this project does offer in this regard is a framework for this research and a set of clues on where resources for this task might be found. The provisional findings of this research suggest that diverse value-aspects of cases are rooted in diverse sets of professional and institutional relations that are operative in the lives of professionals and clients in a case. These diverse value-aspects of cases seem to be championed differently by different professional "types" because of the different ways in which professional practice brings them into contact with patients'/clients' lives. Implicit ethical convictions linked to professional types define patterns of accountability that tend to focus attention on some value-aspects and not on others. Research that explored these linkages in relation to concrete types of cases could deepen our understanding of this aspect of value conflicts and provide tools for understanding when conflicts are grounded in the diverse perceptions of professional types.

Further research would also need to identify typical configurations or conjunctions of value-aspects of cases that practitioners could recognize in their routine practice. This would allow them to assess how the well-being of patients or clients is implicated differently in the various configurations and how this assessment can provide a corrective to tendencies toward bias in professional types. Ethical notions like well-being are not fixed concepts to be defined in the abstract. Rather, they are concrete conjunctions of social relations that take on specific forms or features in defined settings. Practitioners, in dialogue with patients/clients, families and their advocates, are continually making judgments on the concrete content of "well-being." This research would suggest that a social-scheme approach toward understanding diverse configurations of "well-being" could provide tools to help professionals understand and assess the patterns of value relations implicated in the lives of patients and clients. Such a wealth of concrete insights could help them differentiate between their own professional concerns and the diverse goods of their patients and clients.

(3) The third recommendation concerns the *Guide for Ethical Deliberation*. We have presented a first version of the guide and we have "road tested" it with two teams of health care professionals. Clearly, an adequate test of the guide's relevance would require more extensive training sessions to help professionals understand and assimilate the insights and tools. This line of research would need to evaluate the guide and it would need to evaluate the training. In the long run, both types of research will be necessary if the insights proposed here continue to reveal their relevance. We expect that in assessing the guide, researchers will also elaborate on it, develop it and correct errors. In particular, we can envision a development of the self-assessment tool. The provisional results of this project would suggest that further research would benefit from a close interaction between theoretical research and the practical involvement of professional teams.

(4) While this project concentrated on the links between professional types and ethical obligations and commitments, further research needs to probe the possible links between professional types and ethical methods. Deontological or obligation-centred methods highlight different dimensions of ethical cases than do teleological or goal-centred methods. Similarly, rights-based methods champion different dimensions than do context-based, culture-oriented methods. If this research is correct in suggesting that professional types play a significant role in ethical discourse, then research probing possible correlations between professional types and ethical methods could further explain how differing professions and

professional styles focus attention and prioritize values differently. It could also help explain patterns of conflictual interactions among practitioners if professional types were found to correlate with methods that prioritize values in conflicting ways.

(5) The final recommendation concerns the theoretical framework for the research and the links with proceduralist and contextualist streams in ethical theory. While the theory framework of this project is proposed as a means of integrating the contributions of these two diverse approaches to ethics, this proposal remains a hypothesis that has yet to be tested in full debate with proponents of alternate approaches. This theoretical research needs to be pursued.

These recommendations are in no way meant to be exhaustive. In large measure they arise from the research team's awareness of the limits of this project and the steps that seem to be required to overcome them. However, they also arise out of the team's confidence in the benefits promised by the line of research initiated here. It is in this spirit of self-criticism and conviction that the results of this project and these directions for further research are proposed.

Concluding Reflections

Kenneth R. Melchin

The changing face of health care has made the task of patient care much more complex than in past decades. This is especially the case in the field of chronic care. Professionals who care for patients, particular young children, face a bewildering array of challenges for which they often feel ill-prepared. These challenges come from the rapid pace of technological change, the diversity of religions and cultures in our society, the collaborative character of decision making, the restructuring of health care funding, the complexities of our diverse institutions of care and the diversity of citizens' values regarding the end of life. For a period of time in the history of health care in Canada, professionals viewed themselves as mandated and empowered to focus attention exclusively on the physiology of care with ever-improving tools for "getting the job done." But recent decades have seen the meaning of "care" expand well beyond physiology to include wide ranges of social, cultural, philosophical, economic, political and religious considerations. The result, in many instances, is an alarming ambiguity about what the "job" is and what tools might be required for "getting it done."

Health care, particularly chronic care, now involves a diverse range of professionals who meet patients in diverse institutional and community contexts and who encounter patients in multiple aspects of their lives. In one way of another, care has come to mean something quite complex and it has become the concern of teams of professionals who understand their roles and responsibilities toward patients differently. Yet programs of care need to be coordinated and organized so that the diverse parts fit together within a common vision. This means that the professionals must talk together to arrive at some agreement on this vision.

Most of the challenges that have made the lives of health care professionals complex and confusing in recent years are ethical in character. To be sure, not all are ethical in the most obvious sense of the term. We do not usually think of the procedures of hospital bureaucracies as ethical issues. Nor do we usually think of the professional obligations of social workers as ethical issues. Yet this is precisely what they are. Ethics is not restricted to the "big issues." It includes the full range of goals, obligations, tasks, skills and virtues necessary for ensuring the patterns of human cooperation that meet the widest ranges of human needs over the longest spans of time. The "big issues" may command most of our explicit attention. But they are only the tip of the iceberg. It is the whole iceberg that is implicated in the cooperative social structures that ensure the competence, fairness and humanity of programs of care.

This study has moved forward with the assumption that the ethical issues involved in health care will not be handled once and for all by professional ethicists. There will certainly remain "big issues" that will require the work of professionals: issues associated with the end of life and the withdrawal of treatment, issues associated with the equity of resource distribution and issues associated with patients' rights. However, even when such issues are resolved through legislation or institutional policies, they only serve to establish boundary conditions for cases. Within the regions of normal practice carved out by these boundaries, there remain hosts of ethical complexities that are left to the decisions of the professionals in the case. Indeed, even when policy or legislation pronounces on "big issues," practitioners often find themselves wrestling with cases that do not seem to be envisioned by the spirit of the laws.

We suggest that in the normal course of practice, particularly the practice of chronic care, the lion's share of the ethical issues in health care will be dealt with in the day-to-day decisions of professionals. Given the diversity of professions and the diversity of types or styles that have emerged within each profession, this means that professionals need ways of identifying and talking through the issues. The aim of this project has thus been to study the ethical deliberation of multiprofessional health care teams and to develop tools to help them in this task. The chapters of this study present the results of this work.

We began by situating the project in its historical context within the field of bioethics. We then conducted a documentary analysis of published literature related to the implicit ethics of health care professionals. The goal, here, was to establish a typology of the implicit ethics of the principal professions involved in the team deliberations: nurses, physicians and social workers. We then moved to focus on the deliberation process itself. We looked to the fields of ethical theory and conflict studies to develop tools for understanding the deliberations of health care teams and to establish a theoretical framework for linking them with the insights from the study of the professions. We then conducted an initial "road test" of the ideas in an action-research examination of two teams of professionals specializing in pediatric chronic care. A series of case-study deliberation sessions was arranged and videotaped and we analyzed these sessions using an analytical grid of questions developed from the work of the first two parts. The team then developed a *Guide for Ethical Deliberation* on the basis of insights gained from the research. We have summarized and assessed the results of the various stages of the project and recommended lines of further research.

The results have been modest but significant and, we think, potentially quite far-reaching in their import. We found that the professionals do indeed understand their roles and responsibilities differently and that these differences are as significant within professions as among them. We found that the ethical issues that shape programs of care are often held implicitly by professionals in the way they see themselves and their profession. This sense of identity is often not explicitly recognized, expressed or evaluated as ethical. The mere fact that some professionals see themselves accountable for the physiology of care rather than, say, the family, community or religious aspects of patients' lives means that their deliberations will tend to direct programs of care along these lines.

More than this, however, the way professionals see themselves in relation to the other professions will often shape the degree to which other concerns get articulated and evaluated in the deliberation sessions. "Team Leader" or "Manager" types tend to see themselves as responsible for formulating and implementing programs of care and they tend to see other professionals as offering data for their consideration and evaluation. This is quite different from "Coordinator" types, who see themselves as responsible for coordinating the discourse toward a team decision. Furthermore, "Advocate" types often see themselves as charged with the task of defending patients or clients from others who are viewed as uninterested or incapable of placing physiological considerations alongside others within the wider horizons of the person's total well-being. All of this has considerable impact on the process of deliberation leading to decisions on programs of care.

To help deal with these difficulties we have sought to offer professionals basic ideas to help them self-identify in relation to others who see their work differently and to help them articulate and reflect explicitly on the ethical concerns and convictions that function implicitly in their professional lives. These ideas begin with the portrait of professional types of physicians, nurses and social workers that we found reflected in the literature. But they also include ideas on how to think about ethics and how to conduct the deliberation process openly, respectfully and effectively.

We turned to the fields of discourse ethics and conflict studies for insights into how this deliberation "works" when it is functioning well.

We found that discourse has a structure to it, a structure that needs to be respected when diverse and conflicting ideas need to be integrated into decisions that must elicit the agreement of all. What we also found, however, is that this structure seems to have a logic to it that is rooted in a more basic structure, the structure of our own minds. Drawing on the ideas of the Canadian philosopher Bernard Lonergan, we found that discourse on ethical issues seems to move forward in a step-by-step process that involves the four basic cognitional operations of experiencing, understanding, judgment and decision. In team deliberations this involves the team members articulating all of their initial positions on the case, probing beyond these positions to find the deeper visions of the goods or social order that are behind them, evaluating these deeper concerns to find a common vision among the team members that can be articulated as a framework for the program of care, and deciding on action strategies that would implement this vision in the concrete case. Each of these stages of the process are important because each involves a moment of consultation, insight, reflection or deliberation that needs to happen if the full range of questions relevant to the case is to be answered. And, because each of the professionals brings a sense of responsibility for one or another ethical dimension of the case into the deliberation process, all must have an input into the four stages of the process. We found the ideas and skills from the field of conflict studies potentially quite promising as tools for helping team members iron out the difficulties that can arise from the interaction among diverse professional types.

To be sure, a lot of loose ends remain. The ideas presented in this study remain to be tested, debated, tried, developed, verified, corrected and enhanced by further research. Still, we think this further work will be worthwhile. In the short to medium term it may not lead to spectacular breakthroughs on the "big issues" in ethics. But then, if we are correct in our analysis, it is not the "big issues" that present the greatest challenges in the field—it is the day-to-day task of working through the deliberation process in teams of professionals who are confronted with an ever-more bewildering array of ethical complexities in the lives of patients. Here is where we think this study will prove helpful.

One final note: If the most tangible products of research are the theories, methods and applications articulated in research reports, the most profound products are the people who are formed through the projects. This project not only brought together diverse fields of research, it also brought together diverse people with their attachments and commitments to a wide range of theories and methods. The people involved in this project sought to embody the insights and values that we discovered and articulated in the research. We were not always successful. However, significant hurdles were overcome at various stages of the project because individuals remained committed to transcending particular interests and achieving common goals through the discourse process. This commitment to discourse in ethics is at the heart of the work of the Saint Paul University Centre for Techno-Ethics. We hope we have been able to embody this spirit of the Centre in this study.

Appendix A

Database for Documentary Analysis of Part 1

Jean-Marc Larouche
and Tim Flaherty

INTRODUCTION

Before conducting any empirical research through observation of a clinical team engaged in ethical deliberation, we decided to do a documentary analysis from which we could set *a typology of the implicit ethics* of three categories of professionals. The groups or categories of professionals considered are physicians, nurses and social workers—the principal professional players in the field of pediatric chronic care. It is our understanding that what lies behind values and decisions are most often implicit ethics rather than statements of explicit ethics. The goal of the documentary analysis was to clarify these typologies. Our database is the result of the documentary search and the source of the materials.

OBJECTIVE

Our initial objective in forming a database was to provide a resource base for the project's documentary analysis. This resource base was to consist of a representative corpus of literature for each of the professions considered, from which we could draw out the indicators of values, attitudes, schemes of acting and decision making, which form the dimension of our portraits of the ideal types.

A second objective consists in having a database in electronic format available for further research in ongoing work in the dialogue in ethics for those both within the Saint Paul University Centre for Techno-Ethics and researchers from outside the University.

Methodology

A representative corpus of literature for each of the three professional groups—nurses, physicians and social workers—was compiled from medical databases and catalogues by searches using keywords such as "nurse," "physician" or "social worker" and "pediatrics, chronic illness." From this list we consulted those sources available to us in the Ottawa and Montreal areas, and chose on this basis over 100 articles and texts for each of the professions that discuss their involvement in the field of pediatric chronic illness. These texts also included some broader and more general works on the professions and their practice.

The selected texts were first read and notations made of the issues most often addressed and of the indicators of systems of valuing apparent in the writings of the particular profession. A second reading noted indicators of an attitude or an approach toward each of the four specific ethical issues (autonomy, location of care, economics and decision making), which helped form our analytical grid. The notations made in both readings are included in the ProCite database, the bibliographical database software we chose for this project. In addition, any abstracts were included and keywords indicating profession, ethical issue, specific disease or illness, institutional orientation or other related issues were added to make the database searchable for our needs.

Results

We have three databases, Nurse (with 145 entries), Medicine (with 114 entries) and Social Worker (with 107 entries). The Nurse database is larger as it contains general works and methodological texts. Each entry in a database contains all bibliographical information on the texts read. In addition, notes on the content of the text, as well as quotations of varying length, have been included by the research team. These provided the information for the synthesis report, the sources cited in the report and additional corroborative information.

There is a separate file containing a listing of the keywords to assist in database searches. The databases are in ProCite, a bibliographical database system that is searchable on multiple levels of fields individually or severally. It is located at the Saint Paul University Centre for Techno-Ethics.

Appendix B

Analytical Grid for the Action Research of Part 3

Peter Monette
and Tim Flaherty

INTRODUCTION

This appendix presents the grid of questions that were developed for analyzing the videotapes of the case conference deliberation sessions of the health care professionals. The grid is in three parts, each part developed from one of the three fields of literature research of parts 1 and 2 of the project. The first part of the grid, entitled "Implicit Ethics of Professionals," was developed from the documentary analysis of part 1 of the project, "Implicit Ethics of Professionals in the Field of Pediatric Chronic Illness," and was developed by Tim Flaherty. The second part of the grid, entitled "Discourse Structure," was developed from the literature research in the field of conflict resolution of part 2 of the project and was developed by Peter Monette. The third part of the grid, entitled "Ethical Structure," was developed from the literature research in ethical theory of part 2 of the project and was developed by Peter Monette.

IMPLICIT ETHICS OF PROFESSIONALS

Research on the implicit ethics of health care professionals from part 1 revealed a range of types of nurses, physicians and social workers. Each type was shown to have a typical way of viewing the goals of the professions, obligations to patients or clients, relations to institutions and patterns of interaction with patients/clients. The following questions, drawn from this research, guided members of the research team in studying the videotaped case conference deliberation sessions among the health care professionals.

What professional types could be identified in the deliberation process?
Did individuals show evidence of more than one type in the process?

Was there evidence of the typical patterns of ethical valuing in the professional types?
Was this valuing implicit or explicit?

How did professionals of similar types relate to each other?
How did professionals of different types interact?
Was there evidence of authority or power relationships
among professionals?
If so, what was their effect on the deliberation process?
Could intraprofessional or interprofessional alliances be observed?
Were there typical or recurrent patterns of conflicts among specific professional types?

Did all professionals participate in the deliberation process?
Did some not participate or participate very little?
Was non-participation linked to patterns of professional interaction?

DISCOURSE STRUCTURE

Research from the field of conflict resolution offers both an understanding of the structure of discourse and an analysis of the communication skills operative in discourse. The structure of discourse is understood here in terms of the stages that unfold as parties move through the effective resolution of conflicts. The communication skills listed here are a small sample of the tools that conflict research has identified as helpful to participants or third parties in moving through the stages. These questions helped the researchers identify evidence of the stages and skills in the deliberation process.

THE STAGES OF DISCOURSE

Stage	Questions
1	Who initiated the discourse? Who initially described the content of the discourse?
2	Can any positions be identified? Were any underlying issues revealed?
3	Was there any attempt at problem solving? Was there any attempt at brainstorming alternative solutions toward common ground?
4	Was there any resolution of identified problems or ethical issues? Did participants reach consensus? Was there any attention to linking solutions to specific professional responsibilities?
General Questions	Did the discourse follow the normative pattern of social discourse? Did each participant have an opportunity to speak?

COMMUNICATION SKILLS

Was there evidence of active listening as indicated by the use of the skills of encouraging, restating, clarifying, reflecting, validating and summarizing?
Was there evidence of cross talk?
Was there evidence of body language?

ETHICAL STRUCTURE

Bernard Lonergan's four stages of ethical meaning were found to correlate with the four stages in the discourse process developed from the conflict literature. The levels are rooted in the four levels of cognitional operations: experience, understanding, judgment and decision. The researchers found that ethical discourse that respects and integrates the full range of values held by the diverse professionals requires moving through the four stages of operations. This set of questions helped the researchers identify the levels of moral meaning in the discourse and how the participants moved through the levels and operations of the deliberation process.

Level of Ethical Meaning	Questions
Interest Opening Individual Positions	List the full range of ethical issues arising in the case. Which of the ethical issues reflect first-level values (explicit, concrete objectives and desires)? Were there positions expressed later in the discussions? How do they relate to the underlying individual and team concerns that were expressed and affirmed in the discussion?
Social Order Underlying Individual Concerns	Which ethical issues reflect the reasons or concerns underlying the positions taken, the values and feelings that reflect the vision of social good or social order that the parties are seeking to achieve in their desired action strategies? How do they relate to the positions expressed in stage 1?
Evaluation Common Team Concerns	Which of the ethical issues reveal commonly held values or frameworks for common action? How did these common values emerge in the discourse? Did they relate to the underlying concerns and values expressed in the previous stage? Do they respect the integrity of these individual values and concerns?
Action Team Action Strategies	What action strategies emerged in the discourse? Did they relate to the commonly held values? Did the action strategies emerge from discussions on stages 2 and 3? Did participants jump directly from positions to action strategies?

Appendix C

Case Studies for the Action Research of Part 3

Kevin G. Murphy,
under the direction of Hubert Doucet

INTRODUCTION

For the action-research section of this project, four case studies were developed for discussion by nurses, physicians and social workers from pediatric chronic care institutions. The cases focussed on multiprofessional ethical dilemmas in chronic pediatric hospital wards. Ethical dilemmas involving DNR (do not resuscitate) orders, multicultural issues and patient care management were addressed in the cases. The illnesses chosen for the cases included asphyxiating thoracic dystrophy, "short gut" syndrome, nemaline rod myopathy, Duchenne muscular dystrophy, cerebral palsy and cystic fibrosis.

Preparation of the cases involved reviewing literature and interviewing professionals working in the field. Researchers sought to identify aspects of cases that were typically encountered in practice and that would create a pertinent and engaging dilemma for discussion in the multiprofessional teams. In the review of literature in bioethics, researchers found that case presentation varied. Some cases focussed on physiological data while others included psychological data. Some were written for experts while others were written in language that laypersons might understand. Cases differed, depending on whether they were narrated by nurses, physicians, social workers or ethicists. Researchers decided that a broad range of data would be included in the cases for this project and that the presentation of information would follow a format similar to that of a patient's chart. Questions and concerns would be formulated from three perspectives, that of physicians, nurses and social workers.

The first page of each case presents a summary of the illness, together with the central social and psychological features of the case. In order to focus discussion, the last sentence of each case summary addresses a treatment question for discussion by the team. More detailed information is presented in three additional reports, one from the physician(s) involved in the case, one from nursing and one the social worker(s) involved.

The physician report presents basic material on the diagnosis, progression and prognosis of the patient's illness. The social work reports present sociological and psychological factors associated with the patient/client and the family and give some indication of the development of these factors over time. At least three social work reports are included in each case, corresponding to three visits of professionals at various times in the case. They describe social and psychological factors associated with the parents and the child as well as the types of problems they were facing at various stages in the condition and treatment program of the child. They also describe their experiences of the medical treatment decisions, their relations with the health care institutions and the pressures in relationships of the immediate and extended family. The nursing report presents interactions of nurses with the patient and the family at the bedside. Also, the nursing report raises questions regarding the direction of outcomes from treatment decisions and the impacts on the child and the family as seen at the bedside.

The notes from the review of literature and the interviews with practitioners are on file at the Saint Paul University Centre for Techno-Ethics. The following cases have been constructed from the information in these notes. The cases have attempted, as much as possible, not to prejudge the issues. Where data involved conversations with family, verbatim reports are included in the case.

Writing the cases involved (1) literature research, (2) interviews with professionals in the field, (3) writing drafts of the cases, (3) inviting professionals from all three fields to review the drafts for accuracy and realism, (4) revising the cases in the light of their reactions, (5) inviting a second review by professionals and (6) revising and finalizing the cases. All cases were translated into French for the Francophone health care teams. The following four cases represent the result of this work.

CASE 1: JASON FOX—ASPHYXIATING THORACIC DYSTROPHY

The Dilemma

You are a long-term care team in a weekly rounds meeting with a decision to be made about an ethical conflict. The nursing staff want this issue openly discussed among the members of the multiprofessional team, which consists of the team physicians, nurses and social worker. A child with asphyxiating thoracic dystrophy needs an operation for surgical expansion of his rib cage in order to live. The physicians and nursing staff feel the operation should not occur, is "heroic" and would submit the child to more pain and experimental surgical procedures. In essence, the team would like a "do not resuscitate" order from the parents. The parents want the operation for their child; they want all that can be done to be done. The team needs to decide whether they will honour the parents' wishes or not.

Physician Report

The patient, Jason Fox, was born one year ago, and from birth has been a resident of the long-term care pediatric ward. He was diagnosed with asphyxiating thoracic dystrophy at birth and transferred from a small rural hospital to this urban children's hospital. Asphyxiating thoracic dystrophy is a rare malformation of the rib cage to the point where the lungs cannot grow sufficiently to support gas exchange and ventilation. This child is at the far end of the spectrum of this disease. Over the course of the year, the condition of ventilation has deteriorated with unsatisfactory gas exchange even though at this time the child receives almost full ventilation, 90% oxygen, with all other medical supports provided. It is obvious at this time that surgery will be needed to expand the rib cage in order for ventilation and the survival of the child to be possible. This surgery entails a high degree of risk due to the rarity of the condition and uncertainty concerning what will and will not work. With surgery concerning the rib cage, it is possible for excess bleeding to occur at any time and there is danger of infection and pneumonia. Even if this operation is successful, it is entirely possible that the same operation for expanding the rib cage will be necessary again in time. With the success of the operation the child will continue to need almost full ventilation technology, for life, on the ward. The length of Jason's life is not expected to be beyond infancy although a certain prognosis cannot be made. It is the opinion of the medical staff that the surgery may be futile and submitting the child to pain and "heroic," experimental surgical procedures.

Social Work Report: First Report

Received consult and met today with Darrell Fox (mid-thirties), father of Jason. Mother, Sandra, is still in hospital in Summerville, one hour away, recovering from birth. Family is of modest income and consists of two other children, ages four and seven, who are presently being taken care of by neighbours. Father is reporting anxiety over condition of both son and mother. Is coping as to be expected with the shock of his child's condition. Is communicative and expressive of feelings of grief.

At times openly sobbing. At this time feels torn between spending time with wife in hospital, with son in hospital, with other two children at home. Mentioned to him the possibility of having accommodations near hospital for his family to stay when visiting Jason. He was interested and wanted me to look into it. Speaks of feeling guilty and responsible for son's condition even though it has been explained that they, as parents, are not blamed for condition. Any change in their behaviour before birth would not have affected outcome of son's condition. Speaks of fearing that he will not be able to provide child with everything he will need. Questions whether he will be strong enough to respond to the great future demands to be placed on him as the father of the family. Speaks of feeling ashamed and a sense of failure in producing a child with such an anomaly. Mentioned the possibility of joining support group comprised of other parents with chronic pediatric children. He was open to the idea.

Social Work Report: Second Report

Met with both parents of Jason: Darrell and Sandra Fox. Both spoke of the fact that they were devastated by the medical condition of their child. Their hopes and dreams for their child had been shattered by realizing the seriousness of his condition. They continue to express deep grief and guilt since they speak of "catching" themselves reviewing their lives and blaming themselves over things they should or should not have done. They have found the support group of parents that they attend helpful in realizing they are not alone in these feelings. They also spoke of having support from their Christian church tradition and community. They said that they feel God has given them this experience for a reason and they are going to learn from it. They see Jason as a "precious gift of life" that they will do all they can to "care for and cherish." They spoke of feeling a strong religious responsibility to support life. Parents spoke of how they had great fear of the hospital and how it was such a totally different environment for them. They spoke of how they felt helpless at first but how the staff had made them feel welcome and included in Jason's care by slowly training them on how to bathe Jason and operate some of the technology he uses. Parents spoke of how difficult it is to be continually visiting Jason when they are an hour away from the children's hospital. Spoke of looking at houses in the city and the possibility of commuting or changing the places of work.

Social Work Report: Third Report

Family dynamics concerning the relationship between Darrell and Sandra Fox and their other children are really starting to manifest themselves. The parents have discussed with me that their own feelings of anxiety and guilt have been heightened because their other two children are acting out and showing sibling rivalries. The parents feel it is because of the lack of attention and time they are able to give their children while also attending to Jason in hospital. Individually, both Darrell and Sandra have spoken to me about the strain that the past year and Jason's condition has put on their marriage relationship. With all the demands that their family puts on them there has not been much time left for each other and their relationship. Yet both also mentioned that the stress and demands have tested their relationship and made it stronger. Both Darrell and Sandra have mentioned that in some way now their marriage is stronger by supporting and cherishing the "gift of life" given to them through Jason. In some ways they have mentioned that Jason is what gives them the inspiration that keeps them going.

Social Work Report: Fourth Report

After the medical team had approached the family about Jason's condition and the choice of surgery or a "do not resuscitate" order, both Darrell and Sandra discussed with me their shock that the medical team would "give up on Jason like that." They felt strongly that Jason was a gift given to them by God and they should continue to explore all means to support Jason's life. The couple also discussed with me how difficult it was for them to feel "at odds" with the staff over this decision. Over the past year they have developed close relationships with many of the staff and now the tension due to differing conclusions on this decision was very difficult. They felt they had to be true to their own religious beliefs and yet questioned whether these "medical experts may know better."

Nursing Report

The nurses have communicated that they have developed a very close and supportive relationship with the whole Fox family over the past year. Because of the amount of time they spent together over the year, the nurses and the Foxes treat each other like family. Darrell and Sandra have spoken with them of the many ways Jason's condition has challenged their marriage and family life. The nurses have often mentioned how they deeply respect and admire the integrity of Darrell and Sandra because of how they have consistently visited and participated in caring for Jason on almost a daily basis. The nurses agree with the physicians that the proposed surgery, necessary for Jason's survival, is a "heroic" measure. They feel the operation will submit Jason to needless and burdensome pain from experimental surgical procedures. The nurses feel a strong responsibility to act as advocates for their patient Jason by relating and "standing by" this professional opinion. The nurses have expressed extreme anxiety and guilt over holding a differing opinion concerning Jason than that of his parents, whom they deeply respect. They want to continue the supportive role that they have fostered with Darrell and Sandra, but now they find themselves unable to support the Foxes' decision. This has caused the nurses to question whether they are imposing their medical values of "heroic measures" on the Foxes.

CASE 2: FADUMA MOHAMUD AFFI—"SHORT GUT" SYNDROME

The Dilemma

You are a long-term care team in a weekly rounds meeting with a decision to be made about a conflict. The nursing staff want this issue openly discussed among the members of the multiprofessional team, which consists of the team physicians, nurses and social worker. A Somalian infant girl with "short gut" syndrome has been on the ward for three months, receiving intravenous feeding while the bowel is recovering and developing due to the operation she underwent. The dilemma arising concerns the tension and distance that have developed in the relationship between the staff and the parents of the child. The parents are feeling they are being discriminated against by the staff because of their culture and their status as immigrants. The staff feel the parents are not adapting to and cooperating with the hospital structure and culture due to their demanding and disruptive behaviour. The fundamental concern of the staff is that if the parents and staff are not able to work together now, the overall discharge, home care and follow-up plans for the child will be inhibited in the future. It is feared that if this conflict is not resolved, the ultimate "loser" will be the patient. The team needs to decide whether and how they will respond to the needs and demands of the parents.

Physician Report

The patient, Faduma Mohamud Affi, was born 14 weeks ago at this children's hospital and diagnosed with gastroschisis. There was a defect in the abdominal wall and part of the small bowel had ruptured through the abdominal wall, through a very small defect and then twisted on the side. When the baby was born, this group of bowel had not received sufficient blood supply. This particular bowel was not functional at birth and part of it was removed by a surgical operation, which left the baby with a very short bowel—not enough to sustain the child. The baby was transferred from the intensive care unit to this chronic care ward. Here she has received intravenous feeding while the bowel develops and grows in order to provide total nutrition to the child. It is unknown at this time how many months it will take for the bowel to reach this stage. The relationship with the parents has been difficult due to the parents adjusting to Canadian and hospital culture. It is felt by the staff that the time and resources used in attempting to satisfy the demands of the parents would too greatly compromise the resources of the staff in addressing the needs of the other patients.

Social Work Report: First Report

Received consult and met today with the parents of Faduma Mohamud Affi, a 16-week-old Somalian girl. Consult due to frustration of parents and medical staff and an attempt to assist parents and family. The staff related that to them the parents seemed unconcerned about the rules and schedules of the ward. The parents also seemed distant from both the staff and from participating in the care of the child on the ward. Parents of Faduma Mohamud Affi immigrated to Canada from Africa in 1988 with two young boys. Through our conversation I learned of the emotional stress they were under at this time. Parents spoke of their frustration and feelings of hopelessness at this time due to the process of immigrating to Canada, before they received the diagnosis of their daughter's chronic disease. Both have post-secondary degrees and speak four languages but these degrees are not recognized in Canada. They have been forced to take low-paying jobs and at times have felt forced onto welfare. Parents feel happy to be in Canada but also feel extreme guilt because many of their family are still in Somalia, some missing or now dead. Many members of their family want them to sponsor them to come to Canada but they do not have the ability to support them.

Social Work Report: Second Report

Contacted a Somalian case worker with an Immigration Centre to gain a better understanding of prevalent beliefs and dynamics within Somalian culture. "The family" is the central focus of Somalian culture and is very inclusive of extended relations, including great-grandparents, grandparents, parents, siblings, cousins, aunts and uncles. In any type of sickness, the family is the main support and prestige for Somalians. It is considered a privilege to have family members visit you and therefore traumatic when you can't support their visits or immigration. Sickness in Somalian culture holds a stigma of weakness, defectiveness and shame for the person who is sick and the family. Although within the family it is admitted and acknowledged that the disease exists, to anyone outside the extended family its existence is often denied in order to "save face." There are two strong beliefs in Somalian culture concerning the causes of sickness. Sickness is believed to occur in the family when the living members of the family have somehow neglected those in the family who are deceased. It is the spirits of the deceased members of the family that take care of those in the family who are living. Sickness is understood at times as a way of making the living aware that they have neglected the duties or rites toward those who are dead. Sickness is also believed to result from someone in the family behaving immorally. Thus the shame and blame sometimes felt in the family when sickness occurs. If an individual was raised with these beliefs, they may still be believed and haunting even if the individual is now an adult and well educated. Somalian culture was reported as a "chauvinistic" culture where male children are more highly valued than female children. Within Somalian culture there is generally not a strong concern for strict adherence to time schedules. In Somalia there is a saying, "If you chase after the world, you will never catch it—so why bother." Within that culture it is not a concern if someone is "late" for an appointment or meeting by a half hour, an hour or two hours. It is felt that you will arrive where you are going when you arrive there. The time you arrive will be the time that God ordains that you arrive there. Most common religious practice in Somalia is Islam. In Somalia, practice of religion was often suppressed. When immigrating to countries granting freedom of religion, such as Canada, Somali people tend to practise their religion more fervently. This fervent practice is almost as a reaction or adaptation to not having had freedom to practice in Somalia.

Social Work Report: Third Report

During this visit with the parents they related problems they are feeling between the nursing staff and themselves. The husband takes the most predominant role in talking with me. While the mother also expresses her opinion, she often allows her husband to speak for both of them. They spoke of feeling suspicious and cautious with all the staff on the ward at this time. They related feeling that their family and friends were not welcomed and shown respect when they came to visit the child, but were treated with disrespect, especially when they were asked to leave the ward. They related feeling insulted that their religious beliefs and rites that they participate in within their child's room are not welcome or respected by the staff. They felt they were being discriminated against both because of their race and because they are immigrants.

Nursing Report

The nursing staff is feeling frustrated and anxious when dealing with the parents and family of Faduma Mohamud Affi. This is due to incidents on the ward that have created conflict with either nursing staff, the families of other patients or simply the regulations of the ward. The nursing staff are not sure whether the root of the conflict is due to cultural factors, personality factors or destructive ways of coping with the shock and pain of their daughter's illness. Three types of situations that have consistently created tension between the nurses and the staff are: (1) The parents are often late for appointment with staff, either to speak about issues regarding their child or to learn and participate in care procedures that the child will need. The parents will show up late and expect the meeting or procedure to occur when they arrive. (2) Regulations on the ward allow for only two family members to visit with the child at one time. The rooms are shared with other patients and their families and this regulation is to provide for a fair and quiet visiting policy. The parents protest when we will not allow them to bring in more than two family members at a time. (3) Small and quiet religious services and practices can often be accommodated in the rooms but some of the services have created so much noise to become a disturbance and an imposition to the other patients. We have asked the parents to keep such services quiet. There is the similar protest that we do not allow more family members in the room to participate. It is acknowledged that the chapel provided in the hospital is not adequate for the religious practices and services of Islam. The father has been hesitant and not participated much in the care of Faduma on the ward. He speaks more of how he is proud of his sons while speaking of the poor future of his daughter; how she will not have a husband and family. It is questioned whether Faduma is valued less by her father because she is a girl and how this may affect the quality of care she will receive at home, once discharged. The nursing staff are experiencing some inner conflict because they find themselves in an adversarial relationship with the family of Faduma when they are attempting to be of service and assistance. In fact, the nurses are feeling suspicion and contempt on the part of the family toward them. They question how they are helping Faduma and her family in the short and long run.

CASE 3: JOHN MURRAY—DUCHENNE MUSCULAR DYSTROPHY

The Dilemma

You are a long-term pediatric care team in a weekly rounds meeting with a decision to be made about a conflict on the ward. The team social worker wants this issue openly discussed among the members of the multiprofessional team, which consists of the team physicians, nurses and social worker. A 17-year-old male patient with Duchenne muscular dystrophy has been living on this long-term pediatric ward for the past seven years. The care and services available to John through his living on this ward are in excess of what his needs at present require. Other infant patients, presently inappropriately placed on other hospital wards, could be transferred to this ward and benefit more from the services that the ward offers. Over the past two years, the social worker and the ward staff have been trying to place John in another health care setting more appropriate for his needs. Many attempted placements have not been successful due to scarce space and resource availability in other community health facilities. Recently the team has located one quality community facility that will admit and welcome John. Adjusting to moving from what has been his "home" is proving very difficult for John. His parents do not want him transferred to this facility because the resources of the facility are less. They feel that both the level of care and the socialization opportunities available to John would be less than what has been available at the hospital. The new facility would also charge some expenses of care to the parents, which the hospital did not and which they are worried that they will not be able to afford. The team must decide whether they will recommend this transfer or recommend waiting until a more appropriate placement may be found. Judging from past experience, there is no guarantee another placement will be found soon.

Physician Report

John was five when he was first brought to this children's hospital because his parents had noticed an awkwardness and weakness as he walked and ran. Neurological investigations, including a muscle biopsy, revealed that he had Duchenne muscular dystrophy. There is no history of muscular dystrophy in this family; John's parents are not carriers and his siblings do not share his condition. At 10 years of age John was admitted into hospital with pneumonia. The pneumonia resulted in breathing failure and John was put on a ventilator. Attempts have been made to wean John off the ventilator but they were not successful. His disorder has progressed to the point where his respiratory muscles will not recover and he therefore cannot breathe independently of the ventilator. When John had respiratory failure, it was an event that both John and his parents had been prepared for. They and the ward staff were in agreement in their desire for John to receive ventilation. During the time John has been in hospital his condition has progressed. At age 10 he had arm function and still was somewhat independent in his activities of daily living such as writing and self-feeding. By the time he reached the late teens, his arm function had decreased, where he has finger and hand use but little arm use. Yet John has no cognitive impairment and is able to self-direct his care.

Social Work Report: First Report

John is the third child of George and Lisa Murray. His two older sisters are married with children and no longer live in the same province as John and their parents. George and Lisa, both in their early fifties, have retired from farming and have recently moved into the city to be closer to John. John's diagnosis with Duchenne muscular dystrophy left his parents, but especially his mother, with feelings of guilt concerning his condition. They felt that they were somehow responsible, through something they had done or not done, for John having this condition. Even though it has been explained to the parents by all of the ward team at various times that they are not responsible, Lisa has mentioned that these feelings of guilt still persist at times. John had been cared for at home by his parents until the age of 10, when he was admitted to hospital with pneumonia. The care at home was very difficult for the parents since it was a rural area with no respite or additional nursing care programs available. When John was admitted to hospital his parents spoke of feeling both relieved and guilty because they felt they were no longer physically able to care for John at home. Both parents have continued to be consistently involved with his care and his life in the hospital. John has been involved in life skills programs from the age of 12. He has no cognitive impairment due to the disorder and has attended a school outside the hospital. John has made friends at this school and has been able to maintain these friendships.

Social Work Report: Second Report

Spoke with John about his move to the group home and his feelings about the transition. John indicated that he was interested in living outside of the hospital setting. He is seeking a more independent and flexible lifestyle than he has lived at the hospital, with the restrictions it has entailed.

He is not able to articulate what that lifestyle would be concretely. John spoke about both the grief and uncertainty he is feeling in facing the transition from the hospital to the group home. He spoke of how the ward felt like "home" to him and how the staff felt like "family." He related that he had such a strong trust in some of the staff that he felt he could discuss anything with them. John described his tour of the group home and was saddened that he would have to "start all over again" with a new staff, new "home," new school and new friends. The group home is in a different school jurisdiction than the one he had been attending. John was scared that he would not be happy there because, as he mentioned, "they are all much older than me there." He was worried about how he would adapt to life at the group home. John also revealed how he felt guilty for "being in a space that some other little kid needed." Said he feels caught in the middle of something that seems out of his hands.

Social Work Report: Third Report

Spoke with John's parents about moving John to the group home and their feelings surrounding this transition. Parents related that they did not want their son transferred to the group home. They pointed to John's own reluctance to leave what has been his "home" for the past seven years. Parents related how a "human face" has been developed with the staff of this hospital over the years. They know all the staff on the ward and in many other areas of the hospital. With this transition they feel they would have to start from the beginning again with the group home with no guarantee that the same cooperative relationships and intimacy would be developed. Parents were concerned that there is no guarantee that the staff at the group home will allow them the same high level of input concerning John's care that they have received on this hospital ward. Parents questioned whether the staff at this group home would have skills and interest to deal with the needs of a young person like John. John would also be unique as the first person on a ventilator that this home would have accepted. On their tour of the facility they noticed that John would also be the youngest of the residents at the home by at least 30 years. Even though they were assured by the staff at the home that there would be no problems, they were worried about how this home would address John's emotional and socialization needs. They felt John's quality of life would decrease. Parents were also concerned about John having to attend a different school than he had been and how this change would affect his friendships and his socialization. The parents expressed the fear that once transferred to this group home, John would not have another opportunity to be transferred to a more appropriate facility if that possibility arose.

Nursing Report

The nurses have communicated that they have developed a very good and supportive relationship with John, his parents and in fact the whole Murray family over the time that John has been in the hospital. The nursing staff are divided over what should occur with John. Some feel he should stay in the hospital because the group home will not adequately fulfil John's needs for socialization and emotional well-being. Others feel this situation is more a resource issue and that with the current climate of limited resources, John (now a teenager/adult) should leave the pediatric ward and go to the group home. All of the staff have expressed concern and feelings of confusion over what is the appropriate action to take. All are fond of John and express some grief over the possibility of his leaving. Some of those nurses who feel John should leave the ward have expressed some anxiety and guilt over disagreeing with John's parents, whom they have usually attempted to support.

CASE 4: JUSTINE GALLANT—NEMALINE ROD MYOPATHY

The Dilemma

You are a long-term care team in a weekly rounds meeting with a decision to be made about an ethical conflict. The nursing staff want this issue openly discussed among the members of the multiprofessional team, which consists of the team physicians, nurses and social worker. Justine is a four-week-old child diagnosed with nemaline rod myopathy. Her parents have been informed that, in the future, the impairment of the skeletal muscles around the diaphragm would necessitate a tracheostomy and the use of a ventilator. The parents have decided that they want a DNR order for Justine and do not want her put on a ventilator. This decision of the parents has caused some division among the ward team. Some of the team feel the parents' decision should be supported. Other members of the team feel that Justine could be managed and live comfortably with the ventilator and that the parents' decision is contrary to their role of supporting the patient's life. The parents have felt this resistance and team conflict with their decision and have been angered by it. They have asked why they were given a decision to make if that decision was not going to be honoured; they want the DNR order to stand. The team needs to decide whether they will honour the parents DNR order and not put Justine on the ventilator.

Physician Report

The patient, Justine Gallant, was born in this children's hospital four weeks ago. From birth, Justine presented problems concerning muscle weakness. Neurological investigations, including a muscle biopsy, revealed that Justine has nemaline rod myopathy. Nemaline rod myopathy is a muscular disorder that causes respiratory difficulty. There is no cognitive impairment with Justine. This condition confronts the ward team and Justine's parents with the fact that if Justine is to live, she would need a tracheostomy to open up the airway. Due to further deterioration of muscles, this procedure would be soon followed by the use of a ventilator machine if she is to live. With this condition, all other major body movements are impaired due to the damaged skeletal muscles, to the point where Justine will be able to do nothing for herself. The attending physician believes that the child can be managed and made comfortable with a tracheostomy and ventilation. Feels that not supporting the life of the patient, especially since there is no cognitive impairment, would be contrary to the physician's role.

Social Work Report: First Report

Received consult and met today with parents of Justine, Jean-Luc and Carole. It is only the second day after they have received the diagnosis and prognosis of their daughter's condition. Jean-Luc and Carole live and are originally from this city. Most of their extended family is also in the city and they speak of receiving strong emotional support from them. Justine is their first child and the couple have been married for three years. Since they were open to the idea, I put Jean-Luc and Carole in touch with a support group for parents with children with similar chronic pediatric diseases. Couple spoke of how they felt; they were still in a state of shock about the diagnosis of their child. They both at times spoke of things they had done before the pregnancy that they now feel that they should not have done. They feel that their actions may have directly or indirectly caused Justine's condition. At times during our visit, the parents openly sobbed and grieved over their daughter's condition. The parents had been informed about Justine's disease and its effects concerning her ability to breathe. They were deeply saddened by this information and considered her future dismal.

Social Work Report: Second Report

Met with Jean-Luc and Carole today, who were asked to consider whether they would want Justine to receive a tracheostomy or ventilator when it became necessary. In other words, whether they wanted a "do not resuscitate" order for Justine or whether they would allow the methods used to keep her alive. Spoke of how they felt scared that the decision was in their hands and they questioned whether they knew the implications of different decisions. Also related how helpful the physician and nursing staff were in answering their questions. Did not think they were competent to make the decision at first. Thought the decision should be made by the team on the ward. Mentioned the tension that making such a decision caused between them and the anxiety they went through in the process of weighing different factors. Mentioned how they appreciated the support they were receiving from the staff, their family and the support group they were in contact with. Decided that the future for Justine was bleak and that she would have very little quality of life being fully dependent on a ventilator. Wanted to put a DNR order on Justine but concerned that she not have much pain when she died. Spoke of how this was the hardest decision they have ever had to make together and the anxiety they went through in the process.

Social Work Report: Third Report

Met with Jean-Luc and Carole, who were very angry about the conflict over the decision they had made concerning Justine's treatment. They said they felt a cool response from some of the staff and a lack of support for their decision. They mentioned that this response made them feel that they were subtly being told to reconsider their decision. Jean-Luc and Carole understood the concern and principle of some of the staff, who felt their decision was contrary to their role of supporting the life of their patient. Yet, they felt as parents of the child that their decision was also made out of concern for the child and that it should be followed. Both parents were angry that they were asked to make a decision and then seemed to be told that their decision was not acceptable. Their question was "Why ask us to make a decision about our daughter, put us through the anxiety of that decision and then not respect our decision? In fact, suggest that we should change our mind!"

Nursing Report

The nursing staff are split over this decision. The split has caused great anxiety between the staff and poses a threat to the cohesive functioning of the ward team. Some staff feel we should respect and follow the decision of the parents. These nurses agree that keeping the child alive would be submitting the child to unnecessary treatment, considering the child's prognosis and future. Other nursing staff also feel that the treatment of a tracheostomy and ventilation are not extraordinary or necessarily aggressive treatments. Since the child is not cognitively impaired they have difficulty in not applying ventilation.

BIBLIOGRAPHY

Chapter 1—Historical Context: Deliberation and Methodology in Bioethics

Allen, Joseph, L. *Love and Conflict.* Nashville: Abingdon Press, 1984.

Axelrod, Robert. *The Evolution of Co-operation.* New York: Harper and Row, 1985.

Beauchamp, Tom L., and James F. Childress. *Principles of Biomedical Ethics.* New York: Oxford University Press, 1979.

Byrne, Patrick H. "Jane Jacobs and the Common Good." In *Ethics in Making a Living,* 169-189. Ed. Fred Lawrence. Atlanta: Scholars Press, 1989.

Callahan, Daniel. "Bioethics as a Discipline." In *Biomedical Ethics and the Law,* 1-11. Ed. J. M. Humber and R. F. Almeder. New York: Plenum Press, 1976.

————. "The Emergence of Bioethics." In *Science, Ethics and Medicine: The Foundations of Ethics and Its Relationship to Science,* vol. 1, x-xxvi (preface). Ed. H. T. Engelhardt and D. Callahan. New York: The Hastings Center, 1976.

————. "An Interview with Daniel Callahan." *Second Opinion* 9 (1988): 52-69.

————. *What Kind of Life: The Limits of Medical Progress.* New York: Simon and Schuster, 1990.

Carpenter, Susan L., and W. J. D. Kennedy. *Managing Public Disputes: A Practical Guide to Handling Conflict and Reaching Agreements.* San Francisco: Jossey-Bass Publishers, 1988.

Charon, Rita. "Narrative Contributions to Medical Ethics." In *A Matter of Principles? Ferment in U.S. Bioethics,* 260-278. Ed. E. R. Dubose, R. P. Hamel and L. J. O'Connel. Valley Forge, Pa.: Trinity Press International, 1994.

CIOMS. *International Ethical Guidelines for Biomedical Research Involving Human Subjects.* Geneva: CIOMS, 1993.

Clouser, K. Danner. "Bioethics." In *Encyclopedia of Bioethics*, vol. 1, 115-127. New York: The Free Press, 1978.

Clouser, K. Danner, and Bernard Gert. "A Critique of Principlism." *The Journal of Medicine and Philosophy* 15, no. 2 (1990): 219-236.

Daniels, Norman. *Am I My Parents' Keeper? An Essay on Justice Among the Young and the Old*. New York: Oxford University Press, 1988.

Delkeskamp, Corinna. "Interdisciplinarity: A Critical Appraisal." In *Knowledge, Value and Belief*, 324-354. Ed. H. T. Engelhardt and D. Callahan. New York: The Hastings Center, 1977.

de Wachter, Maurice. "Le point de départ d'une bioéthique interdisciplinaire." In *Cahiers de bioéthique*, no. 1, 103-116. Quebec: Presses de l'Université Laval, 1979; reprinted in Maurice de Wachter, "Interdisciplinary Bioethics: But Where Do We Start?" *The Journal of Medicine and Philosophy* 7 (1982): 275-287.

Doucet, Hubert. "La bioéthique, des fondements philosophiques cachés." In *Les Annales du vivant*, 914-915. Paris: Presses Universitaires de France, 1999.

Drane, James F. *Becoming a Good Doctor: The Place of Virtue and Character in Medical Ethics*. Kansas City, Mo.: Sheed and Ward, 1988.

Druckman, Daniel, B. J. Broome and S. H. Korper. "Value Differences and Conflict Resolution: Facilitation or Delinking?" *Journal of Conflict Resolution* 32, no. 3 (September 1988): 489-510.

Fagot-Largeault, Anne. "La réflexion philosophique en bioéthique." In *Bioéthique Méthodes et Fondements*, 3-16. Ed. Marie-Hélène Parizeau. Montreal: ACFAS, 1988.

Fisher, Roger, and Scott Brown. *Getting Together*. Harmondsworth: Penguin, 1989.

Green, Ronald M. "Method in Bioethics: A Troubled Assessment." *The Journal of Medicine and Philosophy* 15, no. 2 (1990): 179-197.

Habermas, Jürgen. *Communication and the Evolution of Society*. Boston: Beacon Press, 1979.

Hamel, Ron. "Books." *Bulletin of the Park Ridge Center* (May 1990): 34-37.

Hoffmaster, Barry. "The Theory and Practice of Applied Ethics." *Dialogue* 30 (1991): 213-234.

Jennings, Bruce. "Possibilities of Consensus: Toward Democratic Moral Discourse." *The Journal of Medicine and Philosophy* 16, no. 4 (August 1991): 447-463.

Jonsen, Albert R., and Stephen Toulmin. *The Abuse of Casuistry.* Berkeley: University of California Press, 1988.

Kondo, Tetsuo. "Some Notes on Rational Behavior, Normative Behavior, Moral Behavior, and Cooperation." *Journal of Conflict Resolution* 34 (September 1990): 495-530.

Kressel, Kenneth, Dean G. Pruitt and Associates, eds. *Mediation Research: The Process and Effectiveness of Third-Party Intervention.* San Francisco: Jossey-Bass Publishers, 1989.

Ladrière, Paul. "De l'expérience éthique à une éthique de la discussion." *Cahiers internationaux de sociologie* 88 (1990): 43-68.

Leininger, Madeleine M. "Caring: A Central Focus of Nursing and Health Care Services." *Nursing and Health Care* 1 (1980): 135-143.

Lonergan, Bernard. *Insight.* New York: Philosophical Library, 1958.

———. *Method in Theology.* New York: Herder and Herder, 1972.

May, William F. *The Physician's Covenant: Images of the Healer in Medical Ethics.* Philadelphia: Westminster, 1983.

Moore, Christopher W. *The Mediation Process: Practical Strategies for Resolving Conflict.* San Francisco: Jossey-Bass Publishers, 1986.

Morison, Robert S. "Bioethics After Two Decades." *Hastings Center Report* 11, no. 2 (April 1981): 8-12.

National Commission for the Protection of Human Subjects of Biomedical and Behavioral Research. *The Belmont Report: Ethical Principles and Guidelines for the Protection of Human Subjects of Research.* Bethesda, Md.: The Commission, 1979.

Ogletree, Thomas. *Hospitality to the Stranger.* Philadelphia: Fortress Press, 1985.

Pellegrino, Edmund D. "The Metamorphosis of Medical Ethics: A 30-Year Retrospective." *Journal of the American Medical Association* 269 (1993): 1158-1163.

————. "Bioethics as an Interdisciplinary Discipline: Where Does Ethics Fit in the Mosaic of Disciplines?" In *Philosophy of Medicine and Bioethics,* 1-23. Ed. R. A. Carson and C. R. Burns. Dordrecht: Kluwer Academic Publishers, 1997.

Pellegrino, Edmund D., and David C. Thomasma. *A Philosophical Basis of Medical Practice: Toward a Philosophy and Ethic of the Healing Professions.* New York: Oxford University Press, 1981.

Potter, Van R. "Bioethics for Whom?" *Annals of the New York Academy of Sciences* 196, no. 4 (1972): 200-205.

Raiffa, Howard. *The Art and Science of Negotiation.* Cambridge: Harvard University Press, 1982.

Ramsey, Paul. *The Patient as Person.* New Haven, Conn.: Yale University Press, 1970.

Rapoport, Anatol. *Fights, Games and Debates.* Ann Arbor, Mich.: University of Michican Press, 1974.

Reich, Warren T. "The Word 'Bioethics': Its Birth and the Legacies of Those Who Shaped Its Meaning." *Kennedy Institute of Ethics Journal* 4 (December 1994): 319-335.

Rothman, David J. *Strangers at the Bedside.* New York: Basic Books, 1991.

Salomon, Mildred Z., et al. "Toward an Expanded Vision of Clinical Ethics Education: From the Individual to the Institution." *Kennedy Institute of Ethics Journal* 1 (September 1991): 225-245.

Sherwin, Susan. *No Longer Patient: Feminist Ethics and Health Care.* Philadelphia: Temple University Press, 1992.

Siegler, Mark. "Clinical Ethics and Clinical Medicine." *Archives of Internal Medicine* 139 (August 1979): 914-915.

Veatch, Robert M., and Jonathan D. Moreno, eds. "Consensus in Panels and Committees: Conceptual and Ethical Issues." *The Journal of Medicine and Philosophy* 16 (August 1991): 371-463.

West, Mary Beth, and Joan McIver Gibson. "Facilitating Medical Ethics Case Review: What Ethics Committees Can Learn from Mediation and Facilitation Techniques." *Cambridge Quarterly of Healthcare Ethics* 1 (1992): 63-74.

Part 1

Introduction

Berger, Peter, and Thomas Luckmann. *The Social Construction of Reality: A Treatise in the Sociology of Knowledge*. New York: Doubleday, 1967.

Bourdieu, Pierre. *Esquisse d'une théorie de la pratique*. Geneva: Droz, 1972.

Bourdieu, Pierre, and Loïc J. D. Wacquant. *An Invitation to Reflexive Sociology*. Chicago: University of Chicago Press, 1992.

———. *Réponses. Pour une anthropologie réflexive*. Paris: Seuil, 1992.

Quivy, Raymond, and Luc Van Campenhoudt. *Manuel de recherche en sciences sociales*. Paris: Bordas, 1988.

Remy, Jean, Liliane Voyé and Émile Servais. *Produire ou reproduire? Une sociologie de la vie quotidienne, tome 1: Conflits et transaction sociale*. Brussels: Éditions Vie Ouvrière, 1978.

———. *Produire ou reproduire? Une sociologie de la vie quotidienne, tome 2: Transaction sociale et dynamique culturelle*. Brussels: Éditions Vie Ouvrière, 1980.

Terrenoire, Jean-Paul. "Approche théorique du champ éthique." *L'Année sociologique* 30 (1979): 57-75.

Weber, Max. "Objectivity in Social Sciences and Social Policy." In *The Methodology of the Social Sciences*, 50-112. Trans. and ed. Edward A. Shils and Henry A. Finch. New York: Free Press, 1949.

Chapter 2—The Nurse as Moral Agent

Abrams, Natalie. "A Contrary View of the Nurse as Patient Advocate." *Nursing Forum* 17 (1978): 258-267.

Albarran, J. W. "Advocacy in Critical Care Nursing: An Evaluation of the Implications for Nurses and the Future." *Intensive and Critical Care Nursing* 8 (March 1992): 47-53.

American Nurses' Association. *Code for Nurses with Interpretive Statements*. Kansas City, Mo.: American Nurses' Association, 1976.

Annas, G. J., and J. Healey. "The Patient's Rights Advocate." *The Journal of Nursing Administration* 4 (May 1974): 25-31.

Annas, George J. "The Patient's Rights Advocate: Can Nurses Effectively Fill the Role?" *Supervisor Nurse* 5 (July 1974): 20-23, 25.

————. "Patient's Rights: An Agenda for the 80's." *Nursing Law and Ethics* 2, no. 4 (April 1981): 3.

Association des infirmières et infirmiers du Canada. *Code de déontologie de la profession infirmière*. Ottawa: Association des infirmières et infirmiers du Canada, November 1991.

Bandman, Bertram. "Do Nurses Have Rights? No." *American Journal of Nursing* 78 (January 1978): 84-86.

————. "The Human Rights of Patients, Nurses, and Other Health Professionals." In *Bioethics and Human Rights*, 321-331. Ed. E. L. Bandman and B. Bandman. Boston: Little, Brown and Company, 1978.

Bandman, Elsie. "Do Nurses Have Rights? Yes." *American Journal of Nursing* 78 (January 1978): 84-86.

Barnes, Corrinne M. "Training Nurses to Care for Chronically Ill Children." In *Issues in the Care of Children with Chronic Illness: A Sourcebook on Problems, Services, and Policies*, 498-513. Ed. Nicholas Hobbs and James M. Perrin. San Francisco: Jossey-Bass Publishers, 1985.

Bartholome, William G. "Withholding/Withdrawing Life-Sustaining Treatment." In *Contemporary Issues in Paediatric Ethics*, 17-40. Ed. Michael M. Burgess and Brian E. Woodrow. Lewiston, N.Y.: Edwin Mellen Press, 1991.

Beauchamp, Tom L., and James F. Childress. *Principles of Biomedical Ethics*. New York: Oxford University Press, 1979.

Bell, Lynn. "Moral Dilemmas in Clinical Practice." *Plastic Surgical Nursing* 2, no. 4 (December 1991): 176-180.

Benjamin, Martin, and Curtis Joy. *Ethics in Nursing*. New York: Oxford University Press, 1981.

Bennett, H. Michael. "A Bill of Rights for Nurses." *Critical Care Nurse* 2 (November 1982): 88.

Bergman, R. "Ethics: Concepts and Practice." *International Nursing Review* 20, no. 5 (September-October 1973): 140-152.

Bevis, Em Olivia. "Accessing Learning: Determining Worth or Developing Excellence: From a Behaviorist Toward an Interpretive-Criticism Model." In *Toward a Caring Curriculum: A New Pedagogy for Nursing*, 261-303. Ed. Em Olivia Bevis and Jean Watson. New York: National League for Nursing, 1989.

Bevis, Em Olivia, and Jean Watson, eds. *Toward a Caring Curriculum: A New Pedagogy for Nursing*. New York: National League for Nursing, 1989.

Britton, LaCrecia J., and Janet D. Johnston. "Dependent on Technology: A Child Grows Up Hospitalized." *Pediatric Nursing* 19, no. 6 (November 1993): 579-584.

Broom, C. "Conflict Resolution Strategies: When Ethical Dilemmas Evolve into Conflict." *Dimensions of Critical Care Nursing* 10, no. 6 (November-December 1991): 354-363.

Burley, Denise. "Theory and Practice of Confidentiality." *Nursing* 4, no. 41 (September 12, 1991): 23-24.

Burt, Robert. *Taking Care of Strangers: The Rule of Law in Doctor–Patient Relations*. New York: Free Press, 1979.

Butler Simon, Nancy, and Debbie Smith. "Living with Chronic Pediatric Liver Disease: The Parents' Experience." *Pediatric Nursing* 18, no. 5 (October 1992): 453-458.

Canadian Nurses Association. *Code of Ethics for Nursing*. Ottawa: Canadian Nurses Association, 1991.

Case, Nancy K. "Substituted Judgment in the Pediatric Health Care Setting." *Issues in Comprehensive Pediatric Nursing* 11, no. 5-6 (1988): 303-312.

Christman, Luther. "Educational Standards Versus Professional Performance." In *Current Perspectives in Nursing Education*, vol. 1, 37-49. Ed. Janet A. Williamson. St. Louis, Mo.: C. V. Mosby, 1976.

Christy, Teresa A. "Historical Perspectives on Accountability." In *Current Perspectives in Nursing Education*, vol. 2, 1-7. Ed. Janet A. Williamson. St. Louis, Mo.: C. V. Mosby, 1978.

Clarke, Juanne N. *Health, Illness and Medicine in Canada*. Toronto: McClelland and Stewart Inc., 1990.

Cleland, Virginia. "Sex Discrimination: Nursing's Most Pervasive Problem." *American Journal of Nursing* 71 (August 1971): 1542-1547.

Coburn, Judi. "I See and Am Silent: A Short History of Nursing in Ontario, 1850-1930." In *Health and Canadian Society: Sociological Perspectives*, 2nd ed., 441-461. Ed. David Coburn, Carl D'arcy and George M. Torrance. Markham, Ont.: Fitzhenry and Whiteside, 1987.

Côté, Anne A. "The Patient Representative: Whose Side Is She On?" *Nursing* 11 (January 1981): 26-30.

Crowley, Margaret A. "Feminist Pedagogy: Nurturing the Ethical Ideal." In *Caring and Nursing: Explorations in Feminist Perspectives*, 189-199. Ed. Ruth M. Neil and Robin Watts. New York: National League for Nursing, 1991.

Curtin, Leah. "The Nurse as Advocate: A Cantankerous Critique." *Nursing Management* 14 (May 1983): 9-10.

Curtin, Leah, and Josephine Flaherty. *Nursing Ethics: Theories and Pragmatics*. London: Prentice-Hall Inc., 1982.

Davidhizar, Ruth. "Honesty: The Best Policy in Nursing Practice." *Today's O.R. Nurse* 14, no. 1 (January 1992): 30-34.

Davies, Betty, and Brenda Eng. "Factors Influencing Nursing Care of Children Who Are Terminally Ill: A Selective Review." *Pediatric Nursing* 19, no. 1 (January 1993): 9-14.

Davis, Anne J., and Mila A. Aroskar. *Ethical Dilemmas in Nursing Practice*. New York: Appleton-Century-Crofts, 1978.

Dock, Sarah E. "The Relation of the Nurse to the Doctor and the Doctor to the Nurse." *American Journal of Nursing* 17 (June 1917): 394-396.

Doell Smith, Laureen. "Continuity of Care Through Nursing Case Management of the Chronically Ill Child." *Clinical Nurse Specialist* 8, no. 2 (March 1994): 65-68.

Dunphy, Ellen, and Marlene Mercer. "The Revised Code of Ethics: An Overview." *The Canadian Nurse* 88, no. 10 (November 1992): 19-21.

Ericksen, Janet. "Putting Ethics into Education." *The Canadian Nurse* 89, no. 5 (May 1993): 18-20.

Fagin, Claire M. "Nurse's Rights." *American Journal of Nursing* 75 (January 1975): 82-85.

―――. "Collaboration Between Nurses and Physicians: No Longer a Choice." *Academic Medicine* 67, no. 5 (May 1992): 295-303.

Frankena, W. K. *Ethics*, 2nd ed. Englewood Cliffs, N.J.: Prentice-Hall Inc., 1973.

Fry-Revere, Sigrid. "A Bioethics Consultant's Thoughts on Caring for Pediatric Patients with HIV." *Pediatric Nursing* 20, no. 2 (March 1994): 177-180.

Gadow, Sally. "A Model for Ethical Decision Making." *Oncology Nursing Forum* 7, no. 4 (Fall 1980): 44-47.

―――. "Existential Advocacy: Philosophical Foundations of Nursing." In *Nursing: Images and Ideals: Opening Dialogue with the Humanities*, 79-101. Ed. S. Spicker and S. Gadow. New York: Springer, 1980.

Gaut, Delores A. "A Theoretic Description of Caring as Action." In *Care: The Essence of Nursing and Health*, 27-44. Ed. Madeleine M. Leininger. Detroit: Wayne State University Press, 1988.

―――, ed. *The Presence of Caring in Nursing*. New York: National League for Nursing, 1992.

Gaut, Delores A., and Madeleine M. Leininger, eds. *Caring: The Compassionate Healer*. New York: National League for Nursing, 1991.

Gikuuri, June P. "The Role of the Patient Representative." In *Bioethics and Human Rights*, 281-284. Ed. E. L. Bandman and B. Bandman. Boston: Little, Brown and Company, 1978.

Gilje, Fredricka. "Being There: An Analysis of the Concept of Presence." In *The Presence of Caring in Nursing*, 53-68. Ed. Delores A. Gaut. New York: National League for Nursing, 1992.

Gillet, Grant. "The Ethical Challenge of Sick Children." *Pediatrician* 17, no. 2 (1990): 59-62.

Graham McClowry, Sandra. "Pediatric Nursing Psychosocial Care: A Vision Beyond Hospitalization." *Pediatric Nursing* 19, no. 2 (March 1993): 146-148.

Guindon, André. *Moral Development, Ethics and Faith*. Trans. Kenneth C. Russell. Ottawa: Novalis, 1992.

Gunby Sweat, Susan. "A Framework for Ethical Analysis." *Plastic Surgical Nursing* 11, no. 3 (September 1991): 123-125.

Gustafson, Winnifred. "Motivational and Historical Aspects of Care and Nursing." In *Care: The Essence of Nursing and Health*, 61-75. Ed. Madeleine M. Leininger. Detroit: Wayne State University Press, 1988.

Haas, Dianne L., Herman B. Gray Jr. and Beverly McConnell. "Parent/ Professional Partnerships in Caring for Children with Special Health Care Needs." *Issues in Comprehensive Pediatric Nursing* 15, no. 1 (January-March 1992): 39-53.

Haines, Geoff, and Stephen Cook. "Left Out in the Code?" *Nursing Standard* 6, no. 15-16 (January 8, 1992): 44-45.

Harms, Dixie L., and James Giordano. "Ethical Issues in High Risk Infant Care." *Issues in Comprehensive Pediatric Nursing* 13, no. 1 (1990): 1-14.

Hofling, Charles K., Eveline Brotzman, Sarah Dalrymple, Nancy Graves and Chester M. Pierce. "An Experimental Study in Nurse–Physician Relationships." *The Journal of Nervous and Mental Diseases* 143, no. 2 (August 1966): 171-180.

Horner, Jacquelynn, and Jann L. Miehl. "The Deontological Decision-Making Model as a Bioethical Tool." *AORN Journal* 54, no. 2 (August 1991): 208-218.

Hull, Richard T. "Dealing with Sexism in Nursing and Medicine." *Nursing Outlook* 30 (February 1982): 89-94.

Hunt, Geoffrey. "Upward Accountability." *Nursing Standard* 6, no. 15-16 (January 8, 1992): 46-47.

Hylton Rushton, C., E. E. Hogue, C. A. Billett, et al. "End of Life Care for Infants with AIDS: Ethical and Legal Issues." *Pediatric Nursing* 19, no. 1 (January 1993): 79-83.

Hymovich, Debra P. "Nursing Services." In *Issues in the Care of Children with Chronic Illness: A Sourcebook on Problems, Services, and Policies*, 478-497. Ed. Nicholas Hobbs and James M. Perrin. San Francisco: Jossey-Bass Publishers, 1985.

Jarrett, Barbara, and Alvery, Denise. "The Nurse as Patient Advocate." *Plastic Surgical Nursing* 10, no. 4 (Winter 1990): 164-165.

Jiricka, Barbara A. "Ethical Perspectives on Client Care." *Saskatchewan Registered Nurses' Association* (October 1992): 26-27.

Jonsen, Albert R. *The New Medicine and the Old Ethics*. Cambridge: Harvard University Press, 1990.

Kelly, Brighid. "The Professional Values of English Nursing Undergraduates." *Journal of Advanced Nursing* 16 (July 1991): 867-872.

Kelly, Lucie S. "External Constraints on Nursing Education." In *Current Perspectives in Nursing Education*, vol. 2, 9-19. Ed. Janet A. Williamson. St. Louis, Mo.: C. V. Mosby, 1978.

Kerr, Janet Ross. "Early Nursing in Canada, 1600-1760: A Legacy for the Future." In *Canadian Nursing: Issues and Perspectives*, 2nd ed., 3-11. Ed. Janet Ross Kerr and Jannetta MacPhail. Toronto: Mosby Year Book, 1991.

————. "Nursing in Canada from 1760 to the Present: The Transition to Modern Nursing." In *Canadian Nursing: Issues and Perspectives*, 2nd ed., 12-23. Ed. Janet Ross Kerr and Jannetta MacPhail. Toronto: Mosby Year Book, 1991.

————. "The Origins of Nursing Education in Canada: An Overview of the Emergence and Growth of Diploma Programs." In *Canadian Nursing: Issues and Perspectives*, 2nd ed., 231-246. Ed. Janet Ross Kerr and Jannetta MacPhail. Toronto: Mosby Year Book, 1991.

Kerr, Janet Ross, and Jannetta MacPhail, eds. *Canadian Nursing: Issues and Perspectives*, 2nd ed. Toronto: Mosby Year Book, 1991.

Kluge, Eike-Henner. *Biomedical Ethics in a Canadian Context*. Scarborough, Ont.: Prentice-Hall Canada, 1992.

Kohlberg, Lawrence. *The Philosophy of Moral Development: Moral Stages and the Idea of Justice.* San Francisco: Harper and Row, 1981.

————. *The Psychology of Moral Development: The Nature and Validity of Moral Stages.* San Francisco: Harper and Row, 1984.

Kohnke, Mary. "The Nurse as Advocate." *American Journal of Nursing* 80 (November 1980): 2038-2040.

Kozier, Barbara, and Glenora Erb. *Soins infirmiers: Une approche globale.* Montreal: Éditions du Renouveau Pédagogique Inc., 1982.

Kramer, Marlene. "Educational Preparation for Nurse Roles." In *Current Perspectives in Nursing Education,* vol. 1, 95-118. Ed. Janet A. Williamson. St. Louis, Mo.: C. V. Mosby, 1976.

Lagaipa, Susan J. "Suffer the Little Children: The Ancient Practice of Infanticide as a Modern Moral Dilemma." *Issues in Comprehensive Pediatric Nursing* 13, no. 4 (October-December 1990): 241-251.

Lamb, Marianne. "Nursing Ethics in Canada: Two Decades." Ph.D. diss., University of Alberta, 1981.

Lazure, Hélène. "L'Infirmière." In *Traité d'anthropologie médicale: L'institution de la santé et de la maladie,* 631-643. Ed. Jacques Dufresne, Fernand Dumont and Yves Martin. Québec/Lyon: Presses de l'Université du Québec/Institut québécois de recherche sur la culture/Presses Universitaires de Lyon, 1985.

Leininger, Madeleine M., "Care: The Essence of Nursing and Health." In *Care: The Essence of Nursing and Health,* 3-16. Ed. Madeleine M. Leininger. Detroit: Wayne State University Press, 1988.

Macedo, Alice, and Lucia Fabijan Posel. "Nursing the Family After the Birth of a Child with Spina Bifida." *Issues in Comprehensive Pediatric Nursing* 10, no. 1 (1987): 55-65.

Maciunas, K. A., and A. H. Moss. "Learning the Patient's Narrative to Determine Decision-Making Capacity: The Role of Ethics Committees." *The Journal of Clinical Ethics* 3, no. 4 (Winter 1992): 287-289.

MacPhail, Jannetta. "Men in Nursing." In *Canadian Nursing: Issues and Perspectives,* 2nd ed., 68-78. Ed. Janet Ross Kerr and Jannetta MacPhail. Toronto: Mosby Year Book, 1991.

———. "The Role of the Canadian Nurses Association in the Development of Nursing in Canada." In *Canadian Nursing: Issues and Perspectives*, 2nd ed., 32-48. Ed. Janet Ross Kerr and Jannetta MacPhail. Toronto: Mosby Year Book, 1991.

Malfair, Amelia. "Supporting the Child with Special Needs." *The Canadian Nurse* 88, no. 11 (December 1992): 17-19.

McDonald, Nancy. "Patient Rep Can Be Viewed as Fiscal Asset." *Hospitals* 54 (May 1, 1980): 44, 47.

Miller, Barbara K., Thomas J. Mansen and Helen Lee. "Patient Advocacy: Do Nurses Have the Power and Authority to Act as Patient Advocate?" *Nursing Leadership* 6 (June 1983): 56-60.

Montgomery, Carol Leppanen. "The Spiritual Connection: Nurses' Perceptions of the Experience of Caring." In *The Presence of Caring in Nursing*, 39-52. Ed. Delores A. Gaut. New York: National League for Nursing, 1992.

Moore, Katherine M., and René A. Day. "Child Care and Family Autonomy: Empowerment Through a Model for Ethical Decision Making." *Humane Medicine* 9, no. 2 (April 1993): 131-140.

Moorhouse, Anne. "A Pilot Study of Bioethics Education of Nursing Students." *Registered Nurse* 5, no. 3 (June 1993): 16-19.

Mordacq, Catherine. *L'évaluation et son influence dans la formation infirmière*. Paris: Centurion, 1981.

Moreau, Denise, and Christiane Larochelle. "L'éthique: un défi pour la formation." *The Canadian Nurse* 89 (May 1993): 44-46.

Murphy, Catherine P. "The Changing Role of Nurses in Making Ethical Decisions." *Law, Medicine and Health Care* 12 (September 1984): 173-175, 184.

Murphy, Jane M., and Nancy E. Famolare. "Caring for Pediatric Patients with HIV: Personal Concerns and Ethical Dilemmas." *Pediatric Nursing* 20, no. 2 (March 1994): 171-176.

Murphy, Patricia. "The Role of Nurses on Hospital Ethics Committees." *Nursing Clinics North America* 24, no. 2 (June 1989): 551-556.

Neff, Jo Ann. "Nursing the Child Undergoing Dialysis." *Issues in Comprehensive Pediatric Nursing* 10, no. 3 (1987): 173-185.

Newhouse, Robin P. "Physician, Nursing, Facility Implications of Informed Consent." *AORN Journal* 57, no. 2 (February 1993): 505-509.

Newton, Lisa H. "In Defence of the Traditional Nurse." *Nursing Outlook* 29 (June 1981): 348-354.

Novello, Dorothy J. "Proliferating Curriculums." In *Current Perspectives in Nursing Education,* vol. 1, 66-73. Ed. Janet A. Williamson. St. Louis, Mo.: C. V. Mosby, 1976.

O'Driscoll, Herbert. "Synthesis: The Larger Perspective." In *Contemporary Issues in Paediatric Ethics*, 91-103. Ed. Michael M. Burgess and Brian E. Woodrow. Lewiston, N.Y.: Edwin Mellen Press, 1991.

Okrainec, Gary. "Males in Nursing: Historical Perspectives and Analysis." *American Association of Registered Nurses* (February 1990): 6-8.

Olsen, Douglas P. "Empathy as an Ethical and Philosophical Basis for Nursing." *Advances in Nursing Science* 14, no. 1 (September 1991): 62-75.

———. "Controversies in Nursing Ethics: A Historical Review." *Journal of Advanced Nursing* 17, no. 9 (September 1992): 1020-1027.

Pagana, Kathleen Deska. "Let's Stop Calling Ourselves 'Patient Advocates.'" *Nursing* 17 (February 1987): 51.

Paier, Geraldine, and Pat Miller. "The Development of Ethical Thought." *Journal of Gerontological Nursing* 17, no. 10 (October 1991): 28-31.

Parette, Howard P., and Phyllis C. Parette. "Young Children with Disabilities and Assistive Technology: The Nurse's Role on Multidisciplinary Technology Teams." *Journal of Pediatric Nursing* 7, no. 4 (August 1992): 237-245.

Pence, Terry, and Janice Cantrall. *Ethics in Nursing: An Anthology*. New York: National League for Nursing, 1990.

Penticuff, Joy Henson. "Ethics in Pediatric Nursing: Advocacy and the Child's Determining Self." *Issues in Comprehensive Pediatric Nursing* 13, no. 3 (July-September 1990): 221-229.

Petitat, André. *Les infirmières: De la vocation à la profession*. Montreal: Boréal, 1989.

Pike, Adele W. "Moral Outrage and Moral Discourse in Nurse–Physician Collaboration." *Journal of Professional Nursing* 7, no. 6 (November 1991): 351-363.

Pike, Sandra. "Ethics, the Law and Clinical Decisions." *The Canadian Nurse* 89, no. 5 (May 1993): 39-40.

Raatikainen, R. "Values and Ethical Principles in Nursing." *Journal of Advanced Nursing* 14, no. 2 (February 1989): 92-96.

Reed, Susan. "Potential for Alterations in Family Process: When a Family Has a Child with Cystic Fibrosis." *Issues in Comprehensive Pediatric Nursing* 13 (1990): 15-23.

Reilly, D. "Ethics and Values in Nursing: Are We Opening a Pandora's Box?" *Nursing and Health Care* 10, no. 2 (February 1989): 91-95.

Roach, Simone. *The Human Act of Caring*. Ottawa: Canadian Hospital Association, 1987.

Rogers, Martha E. "Emerging Patterns in Nursing Education." In *Current Perspectives in Nursing Education,* vol. 2, 1-8. Ed. Janet A. Williamson. St. Louis, Mo.: C. V. Mosby, 1978.

Romaniuk, Camille J. "Patient Advocacy: Survey of Nurses' Perceptions." *American Association of Registered Nurses* 46, no. 7 (July 1990): 15-16.

Schattschneider, Hazel. "Will Nurses Continue to Care?" *The Canadian Nurse* 88, no. 10 (November 1992): 16-18.

Smith, Valerie. "Ethics in Nursing." *Registered Nurse* 5, no. 5 (June 1993): 4, 24.

Stein, Leonard I. "The Doctor–Nurse Game." *Archives of General Psychiatry* 16, no. 6 (June 1967): 699-703.

Sunday Edition with Mike Duffy. "The Modern Nurse." CTV (CJOH-TV, Ottawa). May 23, 1993.

Taylor, Beverly J. "Caring: Being Manifested as Ordinariness in Nursing." In *The Presence of Caring in Nursing*, 181-200. Ed. Delores A. Gaut. New York: National League for Nursing, 1992.

Thurber, Frances W., Janet A. Deatrick and Margaret Grey. "Children's Participation in Research: Their Right to Consent." *Journal of Pediatric Nursing* 7, no. 3 (June 1992): 165-170.

Trandel-Korenchuk, Darlene, and Keith Trandel-Korenchuk. "Nursing Advocacy of Patients' Rights: Myth or Reality?" *Nurse Practitioner* 8 (April 1983): 40-42.

Tranoy, K. E. "Biomedical Value Conflict." *Hastings Center Report (Supplement)* 18, no. 4 (August 1988): 8-10.

Tunna, Kate. "You Are Your Ethics." *The Canadian Nurse* 89, no. 5 (May 1993): 25-26.

Urbano, Mary Theresa, Barbara von Windeguth, Phyllis Siderits and Cynthia Studenic-Lewis. "Developing Case Managers for Chronically Ill Children: Florida's Registered Nurse Specialist Program." *The Journal of Continuing Education in Nursing* 22, no. 2 (March-April 1991): 62-66.

Veatch, Robert. "Models for Ethical Medicine in a Revolutionary Age." *Hastings Center Report* 2 (June 1972): 5-7.

Watson, Catherine. "These Men Worry Me." *Nursing Times* 156 (March 1983): 32.

Williamson, Janet A., ed. *Current Perspectives in Nursing Education,* vol. 1. St. Louis, Mo.: C. V. Mosby, 1976.

————, ed. *Current Perspectives in Nursing Education,* vol. 2. St. Louis, Mo.: C. V. Mosby, 1978.

Wilson-Barnett, J. "Nursing Values: Exploring the Clichés." *Journal of Advanced Nursing* 13, no. 6 (November 1988): 790-796.

Winslow, Gerald R. "From Loyalty to Advocacy: A New Metaphor for Nursing." *Hastings Center Report* 14 (June 1984): 32-40.

Yarling, Roland R., and Beverly J. McElmurry. "The Moral Foundation of Nursing." *Advances in Nursing Science* 8, no. 2 (January 1986): 63-73.

Zuzman, Jack. "Want Some Good Advice? Think Twice About Being a Patient Advocate." *Nursing Life* 2 (November 1982): 46-50.

Chapter 3—The Physician as Moral Agent

Ackerman, Terrence F. "Innovative Lifesaving Treatments: Do Children Have a Moral Right to Receive Them?" In *Contemporary Issues in Paediatric Ethics*, 41-56. Ed. Michael M. Burgess and Brian E. Woodrow. Lewiston, N.Y.: Edwin Mellen Press, 1991.

American Academy of Pediatrics—Committee on Hospital Care. "Child Life Programs." *Pediatrics* 91, no. 3 (March 1993): 671-673.

American Board of Pediatrics Ethics Committee. *Bioethics Reference Applicable to the Care of Pediatric Patients*. Halifax: Dalhousie University, 1992.

Arnold, Louise. "Perspectives for Curriculum Renewal in Medical Education." *Academic Medicine* 68, no. 6 (June 1993): 484-486.

Arras, John D., Adrienne Asch, Ruth Macklin, Larry O'Connell, Nancy K. Rhoden and Alan J. Weisbard. "Standards of Judgement for Treatment (Section 3)." *Hastings Center Report* 17, no. 6 (December 1987): 13-16.

Arras, John D., David Coulter, Alan R. Fleischman, Ruth Macklin, Nancy K. Rhoden and Bill Weil. "The Effect of New Pediatric Capabilities and the Problem of Uncertainty (Section 2)." *Hastings Center Report* 17, no. 6 (December 1987): 10-13.

Asch, A., C. B. Cohen, H. Edgar and A. J. Weisbard. "Who Should Decide? (Section 4)." *Hastings Center Report* 17, no. 6 (December 1987): 17-21.

Bancalari, E. "Care of the Infant with Prolonged Ventilator Dependency." *Journal of the American Medical Association* 258, no. 23 (December 18, 1987): 3430-3431.

Bartholome, William G. "Withholding/Withdrawing Life-Sustaining Treatment." In *Contemporary Issues in Paediatric Ethics*, 17-40. Ed. Michael M. Burgess and Brian E. Woodrow. Lewiston, N.Y.: Edwin Mellen Press, 1991.

Battle, Constance U. "Beyond the Nursery Door: The Obligation to Survivors of Technology." *Clinics in Perinatology* 14, no. 2 (June 1987): 417-427.

Berman, Stephan. *Pediatric Decision Making*. Philadelphia: B. C. Decker Inc., 1985.

Bernat, James L. "The Boundaries of the Persistent Vegetative State." *The Journal of Clinical Ethics* 3, no. 3 (September 1992): 176-187.

Blackman, James A., Scott D. Lindgren and Julie Bretthauer. "The Validity of Continuing Developmental Follow-up of High-Risk Infants to Age 5 Years." *American Journal of Diseases of Children* 146 (January 1992): 70-75.

Blum, R. W., ed. "Chronic Illness and Disabilities in Childhood and Adolescence." *Ethical Considerations in the Care of the Chronically Ill*, 17-27. New York: Greene and Stratten, 1984.

Bränholm, Inga-Britt, and Else-Ann Degerman. "Life Satisfaction and Activity Preferences in Parents of Down's Syndrome Children." *Scandinavian Journal of Social Medicine* 20, no. 1 (March 1992): 37-44.

Brookins, Geraldine Kearse. "Culture, Ethnicity, and Bicultural Competence: Implications for Children with Chronic Illness and Disability." *Pediatrics* (Supplement) 91, no. 5 (May 1993): 1056-1062.

Brownell, Anderson, M. "Medical Education in the United States and Canada Revisited." *Academic Medicine* 68, no. 6 (June 1993): 55-63.

Burgess, Michael M. "Mature Minors: Ethical Treatment of Children in Medicine." In *Contemporary Issues in Paediatric Ethics*, 57-70. Ed. Michael M. Burgess and Brian E. Woodrow. Lewiston, N.Y.: Edwin Mellen Press, 1991.

Caplan, A., A. M. Capron, T. H. Murray and J. Penticuff. "Deciding Not to Employ Aggressive Measures (Section 5)." *Hastings Center Report* 17, no. 6 (December 1987): 22-25.

Caplan, Arthur L. "Imperiled Newborns—Introduction." *Hastings Center Report* 17, no. 6 (December 1987): 5-6.

———. "Imperiled Newborns—Conclusion (Section 7)." *Hastings Center Report* 17, no. 6 (December 1987): 30-32.

———. "Is Medical Care the Right Prescription for Chronic Illness?" In *The Economics and Ethics of Long-term Care and Disability*, 73-89. Ed. Sean Sullivan and Marion Lewin Ein. Washington, D.C.: American Enterprise Institute for Public Policy Research, 1988.

Christakis, Dimitri A., and Chris Feudtner. "Ethics in a Short White Coat: The Ethical Dilemmas That Medical Students Confront." *Academic Medicine* 68, no. 4 (April 1993): 249-254.

Cluff, Leighton E. "Chronic Disability of Infants and Children: A Foundation's Experience." *Journal of Chronic Disease* 38, no. 1 (1985): 113-124.

Cohen, C. B., N. Dubler, M. Genel, J. P. Moreno, M. Mundinger and S. Post. "Familial and Social Obligations to Seriously Ill and Disabled Children (Section 6)." *Hastings Center Report* 17, no. 6 (December 1987): 25-30.

Cohen, Cynthia B., Betty Levin and Kathy Powderly. "A History of Neonatal Intensive Care and Decisionmaking (Section 1)." *Hastings Center Report* 17, no. 6 (December 1987): 7-9.

Coulter, David L., Thomas H. Murray and Mary C. Cerreto. "Practical Ethics in Pediatrics." *Current Problems in Pediatrics* 18, no. 3 (March 1988): 137-195.

Creer, T., and W. Christian. *Chronically Ill and Handicapped Children.* Champaign, Ill.: Research Press Company, 1976.

Culver, Charles. *Ethics at the Bedside.* Hanover, N.H.: University Press of New England, 1990.

Dagi Forcht, Teo. "Compassion, Consensus, and Conflict: Should Caregivers' Needs Influence the Ethical Dialectic?" *The Journal of Clinical Ethics* 3, no. 3 (September 1992): 214-218.

Daniels, Norman. "Chronic Illness: Not-So-Passive Injustice?" *The Journal of Clinical Ethics* 2, no. 3 (September 1991): 160.

Diehl, S. F., K. A. Moffitt and S. M. Wade. "Focus Group Interview with Parents of Children with Medically Complex Needs: An Intimate Look at Their Perceptions and Feelings." Ph.D. diss., University of South Florida, 1991.

Donnelley, Strachan. "Human Selves, Chronic Illness, and the Ethics of Medicine." *Hastings Center Report* 18, no. 2 (April 1988): 5-8.

Douard, John. "Chronic Illness and the Temporal Structure of Human Life." *Business and Professional Ethics Journal* 9, no. 3-4 (Fall/Winter 1990): 161-171.

———. "Chronic Illness: A Problem of Passive Injustice." *The Journal of Clinical Ethics* 2, no. 3 (September 1991): 153-156.

Doukas, David J. "The Design and Use of the Bioethics Consultation Form." *Theoretical Medicine* 13 (March 1992): 5-14.

Drash, Allan Lee. "Juvenile Diabetes." In *Caring for Children with Chronic Illness: Issues and Strategies*, 155-182. Ed. Ruth E. K. Stein. New York: Springen Publishing Co., 1989.

Dubowitz, Howard, Susan Feigelman, et al. "The Physical Health of Children in Kinship Care." *American Journal of Diseases of Children* 146 (May 1992): 603-610.

Eaton, A. P., D. L. Coury and A. K. Richard. "The Roles of Professionals and Institutions." In *Caring for Children with Chronic Illness: Issues and Strategies*, 75-86. Ed. Ruth E. K. Stein. New York: Springen Publishing Co., 1989.

Echenberg, Robert J. "Permanently Locked-in Syndrome in the Neurologically Impaired Neonate: Report of a Case of Werdnig-Hoffmann Disease." *The Journal of Clinical Ethics* 3, no. 3 (September 1992): 206-208.

Fagin, Claire M. "Collaboration Between Nurses and Physicians: No Longer a Choice." *Academic Medicine* 67, no. 5 (May 1992): 295-303.

Fialkov, Jerome. "Peregrination in the Problem Pediatric Patient: The Pediatric Munchhausen Syndrome?" *Clinical Pediatrics* 23, no. 10 (October 1984): 571-575.

Fleischman, Alan R. "An Infant Bioethical Review Committee in an Urban Medical Center." *Hastings Center Report* 16, no. 3 (June 1986): 16-18.

———. "Ethical Views and Values." In *Caring for Children with Chronic Illness: Issues and Strategies*, 81-102. Ed. Ruth E. K. Stein. New York: Springen Publishing Co., 1989.

Fritz, G. K., H. Steiner, J. Hilliard and N. Lewiston. "Pediatric and Psychiatric Collaboration in the Management of Childhood Asthma." *Clinical Pediatrics* 20, no. 12 (December 1981): 772-776.

Gagnard, Liliane. "Le point sur la prise en charge des enfants i.m.c." *Réadaptation*, publication of the Centre national d'information pour la réadaptation, no. 393 (September 1992): 13-15.

Geber, Gayle, and Elizabeth Latts. "Race and Ethnicity: Issues for Adolescents with Chronic Illness and Disabilities. An Annotated Bibliography." *Pediatrics* (Supplement) 91, no. 5 (May 1993): 1071-1081.

Gilgoff, I. S., and S. L. Dietrich. "Neuromuscular Diseases." In *Caring for Children with Chronic Illness: Issues and Strategies*, 183-195. Ed. Ruth E. K. Stein. New York: Springen Publishing Co., 1989.

Gillet, Grant. "The Ethical Challenge of Sick Children." *Pediatrician* 17, no. 2 (1990): 59-62.

Gorovitz, Samuel. "Ethical Issues in Long-term Care." In *The Impact of Technology in Long-term Care*, 23-30. Ed. John M. Grana. Millwood, Va.: Center for Health Affairs, 1985.

Groce, Nora Ellen, and Irving Kenneth Zola. "Multiculturalism, Chronic Illness, and Disability." *Pediatrics* (Supplement) 91, no. 5 (May 1993): 1048-1055.

Grunberg, Frederic, and John R. Williams. "Responsabilité morale des médecins en ce qui concerne la distribution des ressources en soins de santé." *Annals RCPSC* 21, no. 5 (July 1988): 311-315.

Harris, Ilene B. "Perspectives for Curriculum Renewal in Medical Education." *Academic Medicine* 68, no. 6 (June 1993): 484-486.

Heathfield, H. A., and J. Wyatt. "Philosophies for the Design and Development of Clinical Decision-Support Systems." *Methods of Information in Medicine* 32, no. 1 (February 1993): 1-8.

Hensel, William A., and Teresa L. Rasco. "Storytelling as a Method for Teaching Values and Attitudes." *Academic Medicine* 67, no. 8 (August 1992): 500-504.

"Index." In *Contemporary Issues in Paediatric Ethics*, 106-109. Ed. Michael M. Burgess and Brian E. Woodrow. Lewiston, N.Y.: Edwin Mellen Press, 1991.

Jason, Janine, Gloria Colclough and Eileen M. Gentry. "The Pediatrician's Role in Encouraging Parent–Child Communication About the

Acquired Immunodeficiency Syndrome." *American Journal of Diseases of Children* 146 (July 1992): 869-875.

Jauffret, Etienne. "La prise en charge des enfants atteints de spina bifida." *Réadaptation*, publication of the Centre national d'information pour la réadaptation, no. 393 (September 1992): 19-20.

Jennings, Bruce, Daniel Callahan and Arthur L. Caplan. "Ethical Challenges of Chronic Illness." *Hastings Center Report* (Special Supplement) 18, no. 1 (February 1988): 1-16.

Kass, Leon R. "Ethical Dilemmas in the Care of the Ill." *Journal of the American Medical Association* 244, no. 16 (October 17, 1989): 1811-1816.

Klerman, Lorraine V. "Interprofessional Issues in Delivering Services to Chronically Ill Children and Their Families." In *Issues in the Care of Children with Chronic Illness: A Sourcebook on Problems, Services, and Policies*, 420-441. Ed. Nicholas Hobbs and James M. Perrin. San Francisco: Jossey-Bass Publishers, 1985.

Lamarche, Guy, collaborateur. "La pédagogie de la santé: La formation médicale." In *Traité d'anthropologie médicale: L'Institution de la santé et de la maladie*. Ed. Jacques Dufresne, Fernand Dumont and Yves Martin. Sillery, Que.: Presses de l'Université du Québec/ Institut québécois de recherche sur la culture/Presses Universitaires de Lyon, 1985.

Lang, Jean-Marie. "La technique, vrai modalité de la médecine." *Le Supplément*, no. 178 (September 1991): 17-25.

Lantos, John D., and Arthur F. Kohrman. "Ethical Aspects of Pediatric Home Care." *Pediatrics* 89, no. 5 (May 1992): 920-924.

"Letters to the Editor." *American Family Physician* 47, no. 8 (June 1993): 1708-1709.

Lynöe, Niels. "Ethical and Professional Aspects of the Practice of Alternative Medicine." *Scandinavian Journal of Social Medicine* 4, no. 20 (December 1992): 217-225.

Lynöe, Niels, and Tomas Svensson. "Physicians and Alternative Medicine: An Investigation of Attitudes and Practice." *Scandinavian Journal of Social Medicine* 20, no. 1 (March 1992): 55-60.

Malfair, Amelia. "Supporting the Child with Special Needs." *The Canadian Nurse* 88, no. 11 (December 1992): 18.

Mallory, George B., and Paul C. Stillwell. "The Ventilator-Dependent Child: Issues in Diagnosis and Management." *Archives of Physical Medicine and Rehabilitation* 72, no. 1 (January 1991): 43-55.

Marpeau, Michelle. "Conception actuelle du traitement des scolioses 'essentielles' de l'enfant." *Réadaptation*, publication of the Centre national d'information pour la réadaptation, no. 393 (September 1992): 16-18.

Marten, George W., and Alvin M. Mauer. "Interaction of Health Care Professionals with Critically Ill Children and Their Parents." *Clinical Pediatrics* 21, no. 9 (September 1982): 540-544.

McCubbin, Hamilton I., Elizabeth A. Thompson, et al. "Culture, Ethnicity, and the Family: Critical Factors in Childhood Chronic Illnesses and Disabilities." *Pediatrics* (Supplement) 91, no. 5 (May 5, 1993): 1063-1070.

McKenna Adler, Arlene. "High Technology: Miracle or Malady for Patient Care." *Radiologic Technology* 61, no. 6 (July-August 1990): 478-481.

McManus, Margaret, A., and Paul Newacheck. "Health Insurance Differentials Among Minority Children with Chronic Conditions and the Role of Federal Agencies and Private Foundations in Improving Financial Access." *Pediatrics* (Supplement) 91, no. 5 (May 5, 1993): 1040-1047.

Moros, Daniel A., Rosamond Rhodes, Bernard Baumrin and James J. Strain. "Chronic Illness and the Physician–Patient Relationship: A Response to the Hastings Center's 'Ethical Challenges of Chronic Illness.'" *The Journal of Medicine and Philosophy* 16, no. 2 (April 1991): 161-181.

Neal, B. W. "Ethical Decision Making in Pediatric Practice: The Pediatrician and the Community." *Bulletin de l'Association Internationale de Pédiatrie* 4, no. 7 (July 1982): 6-10.

Newhouse, Robin P. "Physician, Nursing, Facility Implications of Informed Consent." *AORN Journal* 57, no. 2 (February 1993): 505-509.

O'Driscoll, Herbert. "Synthesis: The Larger Perspective." In *Contemporary Issues in Paediatric Ethics*, 91-103. Ed. Michael M. Burgess and Brian E. Woodrow. Lewiston, N.Y.: Edwin Mellen Press, 1991.

Orlowski, James P., Martin L. Smith and Jan Van Zwienen. "Pediatric Euthanasia." *American Journal of Diseases of Children* 146 (December 1992): 1440-1446.

Ost, David. "Bioethics and Paediatrics." In *Contemporary Issues in Paediatric Ethics*, 1-15. Ed. Michael M. Burgess and Brian E. Woodrow. Lewiston, N.Y.: Edwin Mellen Press, 1991.

Pallie, W., and D. H. Carr. "The McMaster University Education Philosophy in Theory, Practice and Historical Perspective." *Medical Teacher* 9, no. 1 (1987): 59-71.

Patterson, J. M., and G. Geber. "Preventing Mental Health Problems in Children with Chronic Illness or Disability." Ph.D. diss., University of Minnesota School of Public Health, Division of Human Development and Nutrition, March 1990.

Patterson, Joan M., and Robert W. Blum. "A Conference on Culture and Chronic Illness in Childhood: Conference Summary." *Pediatrics* 91, no. 5 (May 1993): 1025-1030.

Patterson, Joan M., Jeffrey Budd and Darryl Goetz. "Family Correlates of a 10-Year Pulmonary Health Trend in Cystic Fibrosis." *Pediatrics* 91, no. 2 (February 1993): 383-389.

Perrin, Ellen C., Paul Newacheck, et al. "Issues Involved in the Definition and Classification of Chronic Health Conditions." *Pediatrics* 91, no. 4 (April 1993): 787-793.

Persoz-Legrand, D. "La rééducation et le suivi des enfants et adolescents myopathes." *Réadaptation*, publication of the Centre national d'information pour la réadaptation, no. 393 (September 1992): 10-14.

Plante, Dennis A., Seymour Zimbler and Stephen G. Pauker. "A Ten-Year-Old Boy with Cerebral Palsy and Femoral Anteversion: How Much Does It Hurt to Break a Leg?" *Medical Decision Making* 4, no. 2 (1984): 228-247.

Pless, Ivan B., Christine Power and Catherine S. Peckham. "Long-term Psychosocial Sequelae of Chronic Physical Disorders in Childhood." *Pediatrics* 91, no. 6 (June 1993): 1131-1136.

Polu, J. M., D. Foret and E. Chailleux. "Insuffisance respiratoire chronique grave." *Réadaptation*, publication of the Centre national d'information pour la réadaptation, no. 402 (1993): 5-8.

Poremba, Chester D. "Pediatrics and High Risk Youth: A Team Member's Perspective." *Developmental and Behavioral Pediatrics* 1, no. 1 (March 1980): 15-18.

Raphael, J. C., and A. S. Blanc. "La ventilation à domicile dans les maladies neuromusculaires." *Réadaptation*, publication of the Centre national d'information pour la réadaptation, no. 402 (1993): 13-16.

Savy, Jean. "L'ADEP assure la prise en charge de plus de 2700 insuffisants respiratoires." *Réadaptation*, publication of the Centre national d'information pour la réadaptation, no. 402 (1993): 9-12.

Schreiner, M. S., J. J. Downes, R. G. Kettrick, C. Ise and R. Voit. "Chronic Respiratory Failure in Infants with Prolonged Ventilator Dependency." *Journal of the American Medical Association* 258, no. 23 (December 18, 1987): 3398-3404.

Self, Donnie J., DeWitt C. Baldwin and Margie Olivarez. "Teaching Medical Ethics to First-Year Students by Using Film Discussion to Develop Their Moral Reasoning." *Academic Medicine* 68, no. 4 (May 1993): 383-385.

Sherwin, Susan. "Non-Treatment and Non-Compliance as Neglect." In *Contemporary Issues in Paediatric Ethics*, 71-89. Ed. Michael M. Burgess and Brian E. Woodrow. Lewiston, N.Y.: Edwin Mellen Press, 1991.

Shiminski-Maher, Tania. "Physician-Patient-Parent Communication Problems." *Pediatric Neurosurgery* 19 (1993): 104-108.

Siegler, Mark. "Ethics Committees: Decisions by Bureaucracy." *Hastings Center Report* 16, no. 3 (June 1986): 22-24.

———. "Decision Analysis and Clinical Medical Ethics: Beginning the Dialogue." *Medical Decision Making* 7, no. 2 (April 1987): 124-126.

Sigman, Garry S., Jerome Kraut and John La Puma. "Disclosure of a Diagnosis to Children and Adolescents When Parents Object: A Clinical Ethics Analysis." *American Journal of Diseases of Children* 147 (July 1993): 764-768.

Silver, A., and D. Weiss. "Paternalistic Attitudes and Moral Reasoning Among Physicians at a Large Teaching Hospital." *Academic Medicine* 67, no. 1 (January 1992): 62-63.

Simpson, Janet M. "What Do Students Find Attractive About the Practice of Medicine?" *Social Sciences and Medicine* 36, no. 6 (1993): 823-833.

Singer, L., C. Kercsmar, G. Legris, J. P. Orlowski, B. P. Hill and C. Doershuk. "Developmental Sequelae of Longterm Infant Tracheostomy." *Developmental Medicine and Child Neurology* 31 (April 1989): 224-230.

Stanley, John M., et al. "Developing Guidelines for Decisions to Forgo Life-Prolonging Medical Treatment." *Journal of Medical Ethics* (Supplement) 18 (September 1992): 3-23.

Strayer, F. H., C. C. Fethke, T. Kisker and N. G. DeKrey. "Physician Incentives for Shared Management of Childhood Cancer Patients." *Pediatrics* 67, no. 6 (June 1981): 833-837.

Sureau, Claude. "Problèmes éthiques en période prénatale." *Bulletin de l'Association Internationale de Pédiatrie* 4, no. 7 (July 1982): 47-53.

Terborgh-Dupuis, Heleen. "Training of Future Pediatricians in the Field of Ethics." *Bulletin de l'Association Internationale de Pédiatrie* 4, no. 8 (October 1982): 11-13.

Truog, Robert D. "Locked-in Syndrome and Ethics Committee Deliberation." *The Journal of Clinical Ethics* 3, no. 3 (September 1992): 209-213.

Urtizberea, Jon Andoni. "Problèmes posés en réanimation pédiatrique par les enfants myopathes." *Réadaptation*, publication of the Centre national d'information pour la réadaptation, no. 393 (September 1992): 7-9.

Valabrègue-Wurzburger, Odette. "Legal Aspects of Ethics in Pediatrics." *Bulletin de l'Association Internationale de Pédiatrie* 4, no. 8 (October 1982): 5-10.

Venes, Joan. "Pediatric Neurosurgery: Guidelines and Cost Containment." *Pediatric Neurosurgery* 19 (1993): 1-5.

Wahn, Michael. "The Decline of Medical Dominance in Hospitals." In *Health and Canadian Society: Sociological Perspectives*, 2nd ed., 422-440. Ed. David Coburn, Carl D'arcy and George M. Torrance. Markham, Ont.: Fitzhenry and Whiteside, 1987.

Weir, Robert F. "Abating Treatment in the NICU." *The Journal of Clinical Ethics* 3, no. 3 (September 1992): 211-213.

Zaner, Richard M., and Mark J. Bliton. "The Injustice of It All: Caring for the Chronically Ill." *The Journal of Clinical Ethics* 2, no. 3 (September 1991): 157-159.

Chapter 4—The Social Worker as Moral Agent

Abramson, Julie S., James Donnelly, Michael A. King and Mildred D. Mailick. "Disagreements in Discharge Planning: A Normative Phenomenon." *Health and Social Work* 18, no. 1 (February 1993): 57-64.

Abramson, Julie, and Terry Mizrahi. "Strategies for Enhancing Collaboration Between Social Workers and Physicians." *Social Work in Health Care* 12, no. 1 (September 1986): 1-21.

Abramson, Marcia. "Collective Responsibility in Interdisciplinary Collaboration: An Ethical Perspective for Social Workers." *Social Work in Health Care* 10, no. 1 (September 1984): 35-43.

————. "Ethics and Technological Advances: Contributions of Social Work Practice." *Social Work in Health Care* 15, no. 2 (1990): 5-17.

Andrews, Arlene B., Harry Williams and Joe Kinney. "Three Models of Social Work Intervention with Tuberculosis Patients." *Health and Social Work* 13, no. 4 (September 1988): 288-295.

Appolone, Carol. "Preventive Social Work Intervention with Families of Children with Epilepsy." *Social Work in Health Care* 4, no. 2 (Winter 1978): 139-148.

Ashley, Benedict M., and Kevin D. O'Rourke. *Health Care Ethics*. St. Louis, Mo.: The Catholic Health Association of the United States, 1989.

Barmettler, Donna, and Grace Fields. "Using the Group Method to Study and Treat Parents of Asthmatic Children." *Social Work in Health Care* 1, no. 2 (December 1975): 167-176.

Bassoff, Betty Zippin. "Interdisciplinary Education for Health Professionals: Issues and Directions." *Social Work in Health Care* 2, no. 2 (December 1976): 219-228.

Beck, Leah, John K. Lattimer and Esther Braun. "Group Psychotherapy on a Children's Urology Service." *Social Work in Health Care* 4, no. 3 (March 1979): 275-285.

Belcher, John R. "The Trade-offs of Developing a Case Management Model for Chronically Mentally Ill People." *Health and Social Work* 18, no. 1 (February 1993): 20-31.

Bendor, Susan J. "The Clinical Challenge of Hospital-Based Social Work Practice." *Social Work in Health Care* 13, no. 2 (Winter 1987): 25-34.

Ben-Sira, Zeev. "Social Work in Health Care: Needs, Challenges and Implications for Structuring Practice." *Social Work in Health Care* 13, no. 1 (Fall 1987): 79-100.

Berger, Candyce S. "Enhancing Social Work Influence in the Hospital: Identifying Sources of Power." *Social Work in Health Care* 15, no. 2 (1990): 77-93.

Bergman, Anne S., and Gregory K. Fritz. "Psychiatric and Social Work Collaboration in a Pediatric Chronic Illness Hospital." *Social Work in Health Care* 7, no. 1 (September 1981): 45-55.

Bergman, Anne S., Norman J. Lewiston and Aleda M. West. "Social Work Practice and Chronic Pediatric Illness." *Social Work in Health Care* 4, no. 3 (March 1979): 265-274.

Berteau, Ginette. "Un programme de formation continue sur l'éthique en service social: Une réponse à des besoins évidents." *The Social Worker* 60, no. 1 (1992): 64-71.

Black, Dorothy B., Julia Morrison, Linda J. Snyder and Patricia Tally. "Model for Clinical Social Work Practice in a Health Care Facility." *Social Work in Health Care* 3, no. 2 (December 1977): 143-148.

Bodart Senn, Josianne. "Modernité et néo-clercs: À partir de l'image de soi du travailleur social." *Social Compass* 29, no. 4 (1982): 283-295.

———. "Le travailleur social, un néo-clerc qui s'ignore ou se sous-estime?" *Revue internationale d'action communautaire* 26, no. 66 (1991): 89-97.

Bogo, Marion, Lilian Wells, Sharon Abbey, et al. "Advancing Social Work Practice in the Health Field: A Collaborative Research Partnership." *Health and Social Work* 17, no. 3 (August 1992): 223-235.

Bowden, Leora, and Nancy J. Hopwood. "Psychosocial Dwarfism: Identification, Intervention and Planning." *Social Work in Health Care* 7, no. 3 (March 1982): 15-36.

Bregman, Arlene M. "Living with Progressive Childhood Illness: Parental Management of Neuromuscular Disease." *Social Work in Health Care* 5, no. 4 (June 1980): 387-408.

Caplan, Arthur, and Cynthia B. Cohen. "Imperiled Newborns." *Hastings Center Report* 17, no. 6 (December 1987): 5-32.

Chernesky, Roslyn H., and Terry Tirrito. "Sources of Organizational Power for Women in the Health Care Field." *Social Work in Health Care* 12, no. 4 (June 1987): 93-101.

Coates, John. "Ideology and Education for Social Work Practice." *Journal of Progressive Human Services* 3, no. 2 (1992): 15-30.

Congress, Elaine P., and Beverly P. Lyons. "Cultural Differences in Health Beliefs: Implications for Social Work Practice in Health Care Settings." *Social Work in Health Care* 17, no. 3 (1992): 81-96.

Coolidge, Ellen. "Family Therapy and Therapy in the Family: Family Interventions in a Pediatric Inpatient Psychiatry Unit." *Intervention*, no. 89 (1991): 43-48.

Cossom, John. "What Do We Know About Social Workers' Ethics?" *The Social Worker* 60, no. 3 (September 1992): 165-171.

Coulton, Claudia J. "Research in Patient and Family Decision Making Regarding Life-Sustaining and Long-term Care." *Social Work in Health Care* 15, no. 1 (1990): 63-78.

Cristy, Barbara L. E. "Childhood Enuresis: Current Thoughts on Causes and Cures." *Social Work in Health Care* 6, no. 3 (March 1981): 77-90.

Cuzzi, Lawrence F., Gary Holden, Gail Green Grob and Carolyn Bazer. "Decision Making in Social Work: A Review." *Social Work in Health Care* 18, no. 2 (1993): 1-22.

David, Ann C., and Elizabeth H. Donovan. "Initiating Group Process with Parents of Multihandicapped Children." *Social Work in Health Care* 1, no. 2 (December 1975): 177-183.

Dean, Ruth Grossman, and Margaret L. Rhodes. "Ethical–Clinical Tensions in Clinical Practice." *Social Work* 37, no. 2 (March 1992): 128-132.

Dobrin, Arthur. "Ethical Judgements of Male and Female Social Workers." *Journal of the National Association of Social Workers* 34, no. 5 (September 1989): 451-455.

Doukas, David J. "The Design and Use of the Bioethics Consultation Form." *Theoretical Medicine* 13 (March 1992): 5-14.

Falck, Hans S. "Social Work in Health Settings." *Social Work in Health Care* 3, no. 4 (June 1978): 395-403.

Falkenheim, Jacqueline V. "The Education of a Clinical Social Worker: Finding a Place for the Humanities." *Clinical Social Work Journal* 21, no. 1 (March 1993): 85-96.

Feeman, Dorothy J., and John W. Hagen. "Effects of Childhood Chronic Illness on Families." *Social Work in Health Care* 14, no. 3 (1990): 37-53.

Fietz, Margaret. "Children with AIDS in Need of Care and Protection." *The Social Worker* 57, no. 1 (March 1989): 28-31.

Finley, Barbara S., Carol S. Crouthamel and Robert A. Richman. "A Psychosocial Intervention Program for Children with Short Stature and Their Families." *Social Work in Health Care* 7, no. 1 (September 1981): 27-34.

Furlong, Regina M. "The Social Workers' Role on the Institutional Ethics Committee." *Social Work in Health Care* 11, no. 4 (June 1986): 93-100.

Germain, Carel B. "An Ecological Perspective on Social Work Practice in Health Care." *Social Work in Health Care* 3, no. 1 (September 1977): 67-76.

———. "Social Work Identity, Competence, and Autonomy: The Ecological Perspective." *Social Work in Health Care* 6, no. 1 (September 1980): 1-10.

———. "Time, Social Change, and Social Work." *Social Work in Health Care* 9, no. 2 (December 1983): 15-23.

Goldmeier, John. "Ethical Styles and Ethical Decisions in Health Settings." *Social Work in Health Care* 10, no. 1 (September 1984): 45-60.

Guendelman, Sylvia. "Developing Responsiveness to the Health Needs of Hispanic Children and Families." *Social Work in Health Care* 8, no. 4 (June 1983): 1-15.

Gurney, Wilma. "Building a Collaborative Network." *Social Work in Health Care* 1, no. 2 (Winter 1975): 185-189.

Hancock, Emily. "Crisis Intervention in a Newborn Nursery Intensive Care Unit." *Social Work in Health Care* 1, no. 4 (June 1976): 421-432.

———. "The Case of Ann: A Sleep Disturbance in a 3-year-old Child." *Social Work in Health Care* 3, no. 3 (March 1978): 343-355.

Hirsch, Sidney, and Lawrence C. Shulman. "Participatory Governance: A Model for Shared Decision Making." *Social Work in Health Care* 1, no. 4 (June 1976): 433-446.

Johnson, Shirley M., and Margot E. Kurtz. "Implications for Health of Stereotypic Responses." *Humane Medicine* 6, no. 2 (March 1990): 120-127.

Joseph, M. V., and A. P. Conrad. "Social Work Influence on Interdisciplinary Ethical Decision Making in Health Care Settings." *Health and Social Work* 14, no. 1 (February 1989): 22-30.

Kane, Rosalie A. "The Interprofessional Team as a Small Group." *Social Work in Health Care* 1, no. 1 (September 1975): 19-32.

Kugelman, Wendy. "Social Work Ethics in the Practice Arena: A Qualitative Study." *Social Work in Health Care* 17, no. 4 (1992): 59-80.

Lefley, Harriet P. "Training Professionals to Work with Families of Chronic Patients." *Community Mental Health Journal* 24, no. 4 (Winter 1988): 338-357.

LePontois, Joan. "Adolescents with Sickle-Cell Anemia Deal with Life and Death." *Social Work in Health Care* 1, no. 1 (September 1975): 71-80.

Lockhart, Lettie L., and John S. Wodarski. "Facing the Unknown: Children and Adolescents with AIDS." *Social Work* 34, no. 3 (May 1989): 214-221.

Loomis, James F. "Case Management in Health Care." *Health and Social Work* 13, no. 3 (June 1988): 219-225.

Low, Setha M. "The Cultural Basis of Health, Illness and Disease." *Social Work in Health Care* 9, no. 3 (March 1984): 13-23.

Lowe, Jane Isaacs, and Marjatta Herranen. "Conflict in Teamwork: Understanding Roles and Relationships." *Social Work in Health Care* 3, no. 3 (March 1978): 323-330.

————. "Understanding Teamwork: Another Look at the Concepts." *Social Work in Health Care* 7, no. 2 (December 1981): 1-11.

Lurie, Abraham. "Social Work in Health Care in the Next Ten Years." *Social Work in Health Care* 2, no. 4 (June 1977): 419-428.

Mahan, Carol K., Joan C. Krueger and Richard L. Schreiner. "The Family and Neonatal Intensive Care." *Social Work in Health Care* 7, no. 4 (June 1982): 67-78.

Mahan, Carol K., and Richard L. Schreiner. "Management of Perinatal Death: Role of the Social Worker in the Newborn ICU." *Social Work in Health Care* 6, no. 3 (March 1981): 69-76.

Mailick, Mildred D., and Pearl Jordon. "A Multimodel Approach to Collaborative Practice in Health Settings." *Social Work in Health Care* 2, no. 4 (June 1977): 445-454.

Mallory, George B., and Paul C. Stillwell. "The Ventilator-Dependent Child: Issues in Diagnosis and Management." *Archives of Physical Medicine and Rehabilitation* 72, no. 1 (January 1991): 43-55.

Mayer, Jane B., and Renee Meshel. "An Early Intervention Program for High-Risk Children in a Health Care Setting." *Social Work in Health Care* 7, no. 1 (September 1981): 35-43.

McBroom, Elizabeth. "Interdisciplinary Learning in the Rehabilitation Hospital." *Social Work in Health Care* 3, no. 4 (June 1978): 385-394.

Meyer, Margarita, Kutsanellou Christ and Grace Hyslop. "Factors Affecting Coping of Adolescents and Infants on a Reverse Isolation Unit." *Social Work in Health Care* 4, no. 2 (Winter 1978): 125-137.

Mizrahi, Terry, and Julie Abramson. "Sources of Strain Between Physicians and Social Workers: Implications for Social Workers in Health Care Settings." *Social Work in Health Care* 10, no. 3 (March 1985): 33-51.

Montague, John, and Vicki Rosner Stein. "Social Work's Role in Managing Chronic Pain." *Dimensions* (April 1989): 23-26.

Morales, Armando T., and Bradford W. Sheafor. *Social Work: A Profession of Many Faces*. Toronto: Allyn and Bacon, 1992.

Nacman, Martin. "Social Work in Health Settings: A Historical Review." *Social Work in Health Care* 2, no. 4 (June 1977): 407-418.

Nason, Frances. "Diagnosing the Hospital Team." *Social Work in Health Care* 9, no. 2 (December 1983): 25-45.

————. "Beyond Relationship: The Current Challenge in Clinical Practice." *Social Work in Health Care* 14, no. 4 (1990): 9-24.

Nolan, Terry, Inta Zvagulis and Barry Pless. "Controlled Trial of Social Work in Childhood Chronic Illness." *The Lancet* (August 1987): 411-415.

Oppenheimer, Jeannette R., and Ralph W. Rucker. "The Effect of Parental Relationships on the Management of Cystic Fibrosis and Guidelines for Social Work Intervention." *Social Work in Health Care* 5, no. 4 (June 1980): 409-419.

Palmer, Sally E. "Social Work in Home Dialysis: Responding to Trends in Health Care." *Social Work in Health Care* 3, no. 4 (June 1978): 363-384.

Perretz, Edgar A. "Social Work Education for the Field of Health: A Report of Findings from a Survey of Curricula." *Social Work in Health Care* 1, no. 3 (March 1976): 357-365.

Pfouts, Jane H., and Brandon McDaniel. "Medical Handmaidens or Professional Colleagues: A Survey of Social Work Practice in the Pediatrics Departments of Twenty-Eight Teaching Hospitals." *Social Work in Health Care* 2, no. 3 (March 1977): 275-283.

Rabin, Claire, and Dvora Zelner. "The Role of Assertiveness in Clarifying Roles and Strengthening Job Satisfaction of Social Workers in Multidisciplinary Mental Health Settings." *British Journal of Social Workers* 22 (1992): 17-32.

Rapp, Charles A., and James Hanson. "Towards a Model Social Work Curriculum for Practice with the Chronically Mentally Ill." *Community Mental Health Journal* 24, no. 4 (December 1988): 270-282.

Rappaport, Claudia. "Helping Parents When Their Newborn Infants Die: Social Work Implications." *Social Work in Health Care* 6, no. 3 (March 1981): 57-67.

Raymond, Frank B. "Social Work Education for Health Care Practice." *Social Work in Health Care* 2, no. 4 (June 1977): 429-438.

Rice, Nancy, Betty Satterwhite and I. B. Pless. "Family Counselors in a Paediatric Specialty Clinic Setting." *Social Work in Health Care* 2, no. 2 (December 1976): 193-203.

Roberts, Cleora S. "Conflicting Professional Values in Social Work and Medicine." *Health and Social Work* 14, no. 3 (August 1989): 211-218.

Rosenberg, Gary. "The Known and Unknown About the Chronically Ill." *Social Work in Health Care* 15, no. 3 (1991): 1-7.

Ross, Judith W. "Social Work Intervention with Families of Children with Cancer: The Changing Critical Phases." *Social Work in Health Care* 3, no. 3 (March 1978): 257-272.

————. "The Role of the Social Worker with Long-term Survivors of Childhood Cancer and Their Families." *Social Work in Health Care* 7, no. 4 (June 1982): 1-13.

————. "Decision Making and Social Work: Another Look." *Health and Social Work* 18, no. 1 (February 1993): 3-6.

Rudolph, Claire, Virginia Andrews, Kathryn Strother Ratcliff and Dorothy A. Downes. "Training Social Workers to Aid Chronically Ill Children and Their Families." In *Issues in the Care of Children with Chronic Illness: A Sourcebook on Problems, Services, and Policies*, 577-590. Ed. Nicholas Hobbs and James M. Perrin. San Francisco: Jossey-Bass Publishers, 1985.

Sands, Roberta G., Judith Stafford and Marleen McClelland. "'I Beg to Differ': Conflict in the Interdisciplinary Team." *Social Work in Health Care* 14, no. 3 (1990): 55-72.

Schild, Sylvia. "Beyond Diagnosis: Issues in Recurrent Counseling of Parents of the Mentally Retarded." *Social Work in Health Care* 8, no. 1 (September 1982): 81-93.

Schultz, Susan K. "Compliance with Therapeutic Regimens in Pediatrics: A Review of Implications for Social Work Practice." *Social Work in Health Care* 5, no. 3 (Spring 1980): 267-278.

Seiz, Robert C., and A. James Schwab. "Value Orientations of Clinical Social Work Practitioners." *Clinical Social Work Journal* 20, no. 3 (September 1992): 323-335.

Sheafor, Bradford W., Charles R. Horejsi and Gloria A. Horejsi. *Techniques and Guidelines for Social Work Practice.* Boston, Mass.: Allyn and Bacon, 1991.

Sheppard, Michael. "Contact and Collaboration with General Practitioners: A Comparison of Social Workers and Community Psychiatric Nurses." *British Journal of Social Workers* 22 (1992): 419-436.

Sheridan, Mary S. "Children's Feelings About the Hospital." *Social Work in Health Care* 1, no. 1 (September 1975): 65-70.

Silverman, Ed. "Hospital Bioethics: A Beginning Knowledge Base for the Neonatal Social Worker." *Social Work* 37, no. 2 (March 1992): 150-154.

Silverton, Rona. "Social Work Perspective on Psychosocial Dwarfism." *Social Work in Health Care* 7, no. 3 (March 1982): 1-14.

Skidmore, Rex A., Milton G. Thackeray and O. William Farley. *Introduction to Mental Health: Field and Practice.* Englewood Cliffs, N.J.: Prentice Hall Inc., 1979.

Tuzman, Leonard, and Arlene Cohen. "Clinical Decision Making for Discharge Planning in a Changing Psychiatric Environment." *Health and Social Work* 17, no. 4 (November 1992): 299-307.

Wattenberg, Shirley H., and Thomas W. O'Rourke. "Comparison of Task Performance of Master's and Bachelor's Degree Social Workers in Hospitals." *Social Work in Health Care* (Fall 1978): 93-105.

Weick, Ann. "The Concept of Responsibility in a Health Model of Social Work." *Social Work in Health Care* 10, no. 2 (December 1984): 13-25.

West, Margaret, Robin McIlvaine and Clifford J. Sells. "An Interdisciplinary Health Care Setting's Experience with Groups for Parents of Children Having Specific Disabilities." *Social Work in Health Care* 4, no. 3 (March 1979): 287-298.

Williams, Cindy Cook, Neil F. Bracht, Reg Arthur Williams and Ron L. Evans. "Social Work and Nursing in Hospital Settings." *Social Work in Health Care* 3, no. 3 (March 1978): 311-322.

Zayas, L. H., and L. Dyche. "Social Workers Training Primary Care Physicians: Essential Psychosocial Principles." *Social Work* 37, no. 3 (May 1992): 1.

Part 2

Chapter 6—Theories of Discourse Ethics

Ackerman, Bruce. *Social Justice in the Liberal State.* New Haven: Yale University Press, 1980.

———. "Why Dialogue?" *Journal of Philosophy* 56 (1989): 5-23.

Agassi, Joseph. "The Logic of Consensus and of Extremes." In *Freedom and Rationality: Essays in Honor of John Watkins*, 3-21. Ed. Fred D'Agostino and I. C. Jarvie. Boston: Boston University Press, 1989.

Apel, Karl-Otto. *Towards the Transformation of Philosophy.* Trans. Glyn Adey and David Frisby London: Routledge and Kegan Paul, 1980.

Beauchamp, Tom. *Philosophical Ethics: An Introduction to Moral Philosophy.* New York: McGraw-Hill, 1992.

Benhabib, Seyla. "In the Shadow of Aristotle and Hegel: Communicative Ethics and Current Controversies in Practical Philosophy." *The Philosophical Forum* 21 (1989-1990): 1-31.

Castenada, Hector-Neri. "Imperatives, Decisions, and 'Oughts.'" In *Morality and the Language of Conduct*, 219-299. Ed. Hector-Neri Castenada and G. Nakhnikien. Detroit: Wayne State University Press, 1963.

Caws, Peter. "Committees and Consensus: How Many Heads Are Better Than One?" *The Journal of Medicine and Philosophy* 16, no. 4 (1991): 375-391.

Davis, Lawrence. *Theory of Action.* Englewood Cliffs, N.J.: Prentice-Hall, 1979.

Douglass, R. Bruce, Gerald M. Mara and Henry S. Richardson, eds. *Liberalism and the Good.* London: Routledge, 1990.

Gadamer, Hans-Georg. "Replik." In *Hermeneutik und Ideologikritik*, 45-57. Ed. Karl-Otto Apel. Frankfort-am-Main: Surkamp, 1971.

———. "On the Scope and Function of Hermeneutical Reflection." In *Philosophical Hermeneutics*, 18-43. Trans. David E. Linge. Berkeley: University of California Press, 1976.

Gutmann, Amy, and David W. Thompson. "Moral Conflict and Political Consensus." *Ethics* 101 (1990): 64-88.

Habermas, Jürgen. "On Systematically Distorted Communication." *Inquiry* 13 (1970): 205-218.

———. "Review of Gadamer's *Truth and Method.*" In *Understanding and Social Inquiry,* 335-363. Ed. F. Dallmayr and T. McCarthy. Notre Dame: University of Notre Dame Press, 1977.

———. "Discourse Ethics: Notes on a Programme of Philosophical Justification." In *The Communicative Ethics Controversy*, 64-65. Ed. S. Benhabib and F. Dallmayr. Cambridge: MIT Press, 1990.

Hampshire, Stuart. *Morality and Conflict.* Oxford: Basil Blackwell, 1983.

———. *Thought and Action.* London: Penguin, 1990.

Jennings, Bruce. "Possibilities of Consensus: Toward Democratic Moral Discourse." *The Journal of Medicine and Philosophy* 16, no. 4 (August 1991): 447-468.

Kirkham, Richard. *Theories of Truth: A Critical Introduction.* Cambridge: MIT Press, 1992.

Larmore, Charles. *Patterns of Moral Complexity.* Cambridge: Cambridge University Press, 1987.

Larouche, Jean-Marc. "Des sciences morales à une éthique des sciences de la morale et de l'éthique." *Ethica* 5, no. 2 (1993): 9-30.

MacIntyre, Alasdair. *After Virtue: An Essay in Moral Philosophy.* Notre Dame: University of Notre Dame Press, 1988.

———. *Whose Justice? Which Rationality?* Notre Dame: University of Notre Dame Press, 1988.

McCarthy, Thomas. *The Critical Theory of Jürgen Habermas.* Cambridge: MIT Press, 1978.

Moya, Carlos. *Philosophy of Action: An Introduction.* London: Polity Press, 1990.

Odegard, Douglas, ed. *Ethics and Justification.* Edmonton: Academic Printing and Publishing, 1988.

Rachels, James E. *The Elements of Moral Philosophy.* New York: McGraw-Hill, 1990.

Rawls, John. "Justice as Fairness: Political Not Metaphysical." *Philosophy and Public Affairs* 14 (1985): 223-251.

————. "The Basic Liberties." In *Liberty, Equality, and Law: Selected Tanner Lectures on Moral Philosophy*, 3-87. Ed. S. McMurrin. Salt Lake City: University of Utah Press, 1987.

————. "The Idea of an Overlapping Consensus." *The Oxford Journal of Legal Studies* 7 (1987): 1-25.

Ricoeur, Paul. "Ethics and Culture: Habermas and Gadamer in Dialogue." *Philosophy Today* 17 (1973): 153-165.

————. "Hermeneutics and the Critique of Ideology." In *Hermeneutics and the Human Sciences*, 63-100. Ed. and trans. J. B. Thompson. Cambridge: Cambridge University Press, 1982.

————. "Avant la loi morale: L'éthique." In *Encyclopaedia Universalis*, vol. 22, 42-45. Paris: Encyclopaedia Universalis, 1985.

————. "Le juste entre le bon et le légal." *Esprit*, no. 174 (September 1991): 5-21.

Sandel, Michael. *Liberalism and the Limits of Justice*. Cambridge: Cambridge University Press, 1982.

Sauer, James B. "Values, Transactions, and Consensus." Ottawa: Saint Paul University Centre for Techno-Ethics, 1992.

Tong, Rosemarie. "The Epistemology and Ethics of Consensus: Uses and Misuses of 'Ethical' Experts." *The Journal of Medicine and Philosophy* 16, no. 4 (1991): 409-426.

Williams, Bernard. "Conflicts of Value." In *Moral Luck: Philosophical Papers, 1973-1980*, 71-82. Cambridge: Cambridge University Press, 1981.

Chapter 7—The Cognitional Theory of Bernard Lonergan and the Structure of Ethical Deliberation

Byrne, Patrick H. "Jane Jacobs and the Common Good." In *Ethics in Making a Living*, 169-189. Ed. Fred Lawrence. Atlanta: Scholars Press, 1989.

———. "'Ressentiment' and the Preferential Option for the Poor." *Theological Studies* 54 (1993): 214-241.

Cassidy, Joseph P. *Extending Bernard Lonergan's Ethics*. Ph.D. diss., Saint Paul University, Ottawa, 1995.

Conn, Walter E. *Conversion: Development and Self-Transcendence*. Birmingham: Religious Education Press, 1981.

Crowe, Frederick. "An Exploration of Lonergan's New Notion of Value." *Science et Esprit* 29 (1977): 123-143.

———. "An Expansion of Lonergan's Notion of Value." In *Lonergan Workshop*, 35-57. Ed. Fred Lawrence. Atlanta: Scholars Press, 1988.

Crysdale, Cynthia. "Revisioning Natural Law: From the Classicist Paradigm to Emergent Probability." *Theological Studies* 56 (1995): 464-484.

Daly, Herman, and John B. Cobb, Jr. *For the Common Good*. Boston: Beacon Press, 1989.

Happel, Stephen, and James J. Walter. *Conversion and Discipleship*. Philadelphia: Fortress Press, 1986.

Lawrence, Fred. "The Fragility of Consciousness: Lonergan and the Postmodern Concern for the Other." *Theological Studies* 54 (1993): 55-94.

Lonergan, Bernard. *Method in Theology*. New York: Herder and Herder, 1972.

———. *Collected Works of Bernard Lonergan*, vol. 3, *Insight: A Study of Human Understanding*. Ed. F. E. Crowe and Robert M. Doran. Toronto: University of Toronto Press, 1992; orig. New York: Longman, 1957.

McShane, Philip. *Randomness, Statistics and Emergence*. Dublin: Gill and Macmillan, 1970.

————. *Wealth of Self and Wealth of Nations*. Hicksville, N.Y.: Exposition Press, 1975.

Melchin, Kenneth R. *History, Ethics, and Emergent Probability*. Lanham, Md.: University Press of America, 1987.

————. "Moral Knowledge and the Structure of Cooperative Living." *Theological Studies* 52 (September 1991): 495-523.

————. "Economics, Ethics, and the Structure of Social Living." *Humanomics* 10, no. 3 (1994): 21-57.

————. "Pluralism, Conflict, and the Structure of the Public Good." In *The Promise of Critical Theology: Essays in Honour of Charles Davis*, 75-92. Ed. Marc Lalonde. Waterloo, Ont.: Wilfrid Laurier University Press, 1995.

————. *Living with Other People: An Introduction to Christian Ethics Based on Bernard Lonergan*. Ottawa: Novalis; Collegeville: Liturgical Press, 1998.

Picard, Cheryl A. *Campus Mediation Training Manual*. Ottawa: Carleton University Press, 1993.

————. *Mediating Interpersonal and Small Group Conflicts*. Ottawa: Golden Dog Press, 1998.

Vertin, Michael. "Judgments of Value for the Later Lonergan." *Method: Journal of Lonergan Studies* 13 (Fall 1995): 221-248.

Walzer, Michael. *Spheres of Justice*. New York: Basic Books, 1983.

Chapter 8—Value Conflicts in Health Care Teams

Abbott, A. *The System of Professions: An Essay on the Division of Expert Labor*. University of Chicago Press: Chicago, 1988.

American Hospital Association, Special Committee on Biomedical Ethics. "Values in Conflict: Resolving Ethical Issues in Hospital Care." *American Hospital Association* (1985): 67-74.

Arkes, Hal R., and Kenneth R. Hammond. *Judgment and Decision Making: An Interdisciplinary Reader*. Cambridge: Cambridge University Press, 1986.

Aubert, Velhelm. "Competition and Dissensus: Two Types of Conflict and Conflict Resolution." *Journal of Conflict Resolution* 7, no. 1 (1963): 26-42.

Avery, Michel, Brian Auvine, Barbara Streibel and Lonnie Weiss. *Building United Judgment: A Handbook for Consensus Decision Making.* Madison, Wisc.: The Centre for Conflict Resolution, 1981.

Avruch, K., and P. W. Black. "Ideas of Human Nature in Contemporary Conflict Resolution Theory." *Negotiation Journal* 6, no. 3 (1990): 221-228.

Bartunek, J. M., and R. D. Reid. "The Role of Conflict in a Second Order Change Attempt." In *Hidden Conflict in Organizations: Uncovering Behind-the-Scenes Disputes*, 116-142. Ed. D. M. Kolb and J. M. Bartunek. Newbury Park, Calif.: Sage Publications, 1992.

Bisno, Herb. *Managing Conflict.* Newbury Park, Calif.: Sage Publications, 1988.

Brett, Jeanne M. "Negotiating Group Decisions." *Negotiation Journal* 7 (1991): 291-310.

Broom, C. "Conflict Resolution Strategies: When Ethical Dilemmas Evolve into Conflict." *Dimensions of Critical Care Nursing* 10, no. 6 (November-December 1991): 354-363.

Building Consensus for a Sustainable Future: Guiding Principles, An Initiative Undertaken by Canadian Round Tables, August 1993.

Burt, Robert. *Taking Care of Strangers: The Rule of Law in Doctor–Patient Relations.* New York: Free Press, 1979.

Burton, John. *Conflict: Resolution and Prevention.* New York: St. Martin's Press, 1990.

Burton, John, and Frank Dukes. *Conflict: Practices in Management, Settlement and Resolution.* New York: St. Martin's Press, 1990.

Bush, Robert Baruch, and Joseph Folger. *The Promise of Mediation: Responding to Conflict Through Empowerment and Recognition.* San Francisco: Jossey-Bass Publishers, 1994.

Carpenter, Susan L., and W. J. D. Kennedy. *Managing Public Disputes: A Practical Guide to Handling Conflict and Reaching Agreements.* San Francisco: Jossey-Bass Publishers, 1988.

Case, Nancy K. "Substituted Judgment in the Pediatric Health Care Setting." *Issues in Comprehensive Pediatric Nursing* 11, no. 5-6 (1988): 303-312.

Colosi, Thomas. "A Model for Negotiation and Mediation." In *Conflict Management and Problem Solving*, 86-99. Ed. J. D. Sandole and Ingrid Sandole-Staroste. New York: New York University Press, 1987.

Dahl, J. G., and P. K. Kienast. "The Effect of Payoff Matrix Induced Competition on the Creation of Value in Negotiation." In *Theory and Research in Conflict Management*, 77-85. Ed. M. A. Rahim. New York: Praeger, 1990.

Donohue, William A. "Criteria for Developing Communication Theory in Mediation." In *Managing Conflict: An Interdisciplinary Approach*, 71-82. Ed. M. A. Rahim. New York: Praeger, 1989.

Druckman, Daniel, B. J. Broome and S. H. Korper. "Value Differences and Conflict Resolution: Facilitation or Delinking?" *Journal of Conflict Resolution* 32, no. 3 (September 1988): 489-510.

Druckman, Daniel, R. Rozelle and K. Zechmeister. "Conflict of Interest and Value Dissensus: Two Perspectives." In *Negotiation: Social-psychological Perspectives*, 105-131. Ed. Daniel Druckman. Newbury Park, Calif.: Sage Publications, 1977.

Druckman, Daniel, and K. Zechmeister. "Conflict of Interest and Value Dissensus: Propositions in the Sociology of Conflict." *Human Relations* 26, no. 4 (1973): 449-466.

Dubinskas, F. A. "Culture and Conflict: The Cultural Roots of Discord." In *Hidden Conflict in Organizations: Uncovering Behind-the-Scenes Disputes*, 187-208. Ed. D. M. Kolb and J. M. Bartunek. Newbury Park, Calif.: Sage Publications, 1992.

Dubler Neveloff, Nancy, and Leonard J. Marcus. *Mediating Bioethical Disputes*. New York: United Hospital Fund of New York, 1994.

Dukes, Frank. "Public Conflict Resolution: A Transformative Approach." *Negotiation Journal* 9, no. 1 (1993): 45-57.

Fandetti, D. V., and J. Goldmeier. "Social Workers as Culture Mediators in Health Care Settings." *Health and Social Work* 13, no. 3 (1988): 171-179.

Felstiner, W. L. F., R. L. Abel and A. Sarat. "The Emergence and Transformation of Disputes: Naming, Blaming and Claiming." *Law and Society Review* 15 (1981): 631-654.

Fisher, Roger, and William Ury. *Getting to Yes: Negotiating Agreement Without Giving In.* Boston: Houghton Mifflin Company, 1981.

Fisher, Ron J., and L. Keashly. "Third Party Interventions in Intergroup Conflict: Consultation Is *Not* Mediation." *Negotiation Journal* 4, no. 4 (1988): 381-393.

Folger, Joseph P., Marshall Scott Poole and Randall K. Stutman. *Working Through Conflict: Strategies for Relationships, Groups and Organizations*, 2nd ed. New York: Harper Collins College Publishers, 1993.

Friedman, R. A. "The Culture of Mediation: Private Understandings in the Context of Public Conflict." In *Hidden Conflict in Organizations: Uncovering Behind-the-Scenes Disputes*, 143-164. Ed. D. M. Kolb and J. M. Bartunek. Newbury Park, Calif.: Sage Publications, 1992.

Friedman, R. A., and J. Podoiny. "Differentiation of Boundary Spanning Roles: Labor Negotiations and Implications for Role Conflict." *Administrative Science Quarterly* 37, no. 1 (1992): 28-47.

Frohock, Fred. "Reasoning and Intractability." In *Intractable Conflicts and Their Transformation*, 13-24. Ed. Louis Kriesberg, Terrell A. Northrup and Stuart J. Thorson. New York: Syracuse University Press, 1989.

Fuller, Rex M., William D. Kimsey and Bruce C. McKinney. "Mediator Neutrality and Storytelling Order." *Mediation Quarterly* 10, no. 2 (1992): 187-192.

Gibson, D. "Theory and Strategies for Resolving Conflict." *Occupational Therapy in Mental Health* 5, no. 4 (1986): 47-64.

Gralnick, A. "Conflict Resolution and Inhospital Therapeutic Process." *Psychiatric Journal of the University of Ottawa* 12, no. 1 (1987): 21-25.

Grodin, M. A., and L. A. Burton. "Context and Process in Medical Ethics: The Contribution of Family-Systems Theory." *Family Systems Medicine* 6, no. 4 (1988): 421-438.

Habermas, Jürgen. *Moral Consciousness and Communicative Action.* Trans. C. Lenhardt and S. W. Nicholsen. Cambridge: MIT Press, 1990.

Hayes, C. L., B. Soniat and H. Burr. "Value Conflict and Resolution in Forcing Services on 'At Risk' Community-Based Older Adults." *Clinical Gerontologist* 4, no. 3 (1986): 41-48.

Helm, B., and A. M. Moore. "Dispute Resolution in the *Psychological Abstracts*: Publication Patterns in 1990 and 1991." *Mediation Quarterly* 10, no. 2 (1992): 213-223.

Helm, B., S. Odom and J. Wright. "Publication Patterns in the Early Years: Dispute Resolution in the *Psychological Abstracts*, 1980-1985." *Mediation Quarterly* 9, no. 1 (1992): 87-103.

Helm, B., and J. K. Wright. "Publication Patterns in the Growth Years: Dispute Resolution in the *Psychological Abstracts*, 1986-1989." *Mediation Quarterly* 9, no. 3 (1992): 275-294.

Hundert, E. "A Model for Ethical Problem Solving in Medicine, with Practical Applications." *American Journal of Psychiatry* 144, no.7 (1987): 839-846.

Hunter, Susan. "The Roots of Environmental Conflict in the Tahoe Basin." In *Intractable Conflicts and Their Transformation*, 25-40. Ed. Louis Kriesberg, Terrell A. Northrup and Stuart J. Thorson. New York: Syracuse University Press, 1989.

Jandt, Fred E., and P. Gillette. *Win-Win Negotiating: Turning Conflict into Agreement.* New York: John Wiley and Sons, 1985.

Jonsen, A., M. Siegler and W. Winslade. *Clinical Ethics,* 2nd ed. New York: Macmillan, 1986.

Joseph, M. V., and A. P. Conrad. "Social Work Influence on Interdisciplinary Ethical Decision Making in Health Care Settings." *Health and Social Work* 14, no. 1 (February 1989): 22-30.

Kinnier, T. "Development of a Values Conflict Resolution Assessment." *Journal of Counselling Psychology* 34, no. 1 (1987): 31-37.

Kolb, Deborah M. *The Mediators.* Cambridge: MIT Press, 1983.

Kolb, Deborah M., and L. L. Putnam. "Introduction: The Dialectics of Disputing." In *Hidden Conflict in Organizations: Uncovering Behind-the-Scenes Disputes*, 1-31. Ed. D. M. Kolb and J. M. Bartunek. Newbury Park, Calif.: Sage Publications, 1992.

Kolb, Deborah M., and S. S. Silbey. "Enhancing the Capacity of Organizations to Deal with Disputes." *Negotiation Journal* 6, no. 4 (1990): 297-304.

Kressel, Kenneth, and Dean G. Pruitt. "Themes in the Mediation of Social Conflict." *Journal of Social Issues* 41, no. 2 (1985): 179-198.

Kressel, Kenneth, Dean G. Pruitt and Associates, eds. *Mediation Research: The Process and Effectiveness of Third-Party Intervention.* San Francisco: Jossey-Bass Publishers, 1989.

Kriesberg, Louis, Terrell A. Northrup and Stuart J. Thorson, eds. *Intractable Conflicts and Their Transformation.* New York: Syracuse University Press, 1989.

Laue, J. "The Emergence and Institutionalization of Third Party Roles in Conflict." In *Conflict Management and Problem Solving*, 17-29. Ed. J. D. Sandole and Ingrid Sandole-Staroste. New York: New York University Press, 1987.

Lewicki, R. J., and J. A. Litterer. *Negotiation.* Homewood, Ill.: Richard D. Irwin Inc., 1985.

Maciunas, K. A., and A. H. Moss. "Learning the Patient's Narrative to Determine Decision-Making Capacity: The Role of Ethics Committees." *The Journal of Clinical Ethics* 3, no. 4 (Winter 1992): 287-289.

Martin, J. A. "The Suppression of Gender Conflict in Organizations." In *Hidden Conflict in Organizations: Uncovering Behind-the-Scenes Disputes*, 165-186. Ed. D. M. Kolb and J. M. Bartunek. Newbury Park, Calif.: Sage Publications, 1992.

Mather, L., and B. Yngvesson. "Language, Audience and the Transformation of Disputes." *Law and Society* 15, no. 3-4 (1980-1981): 775-821.

Mika, H. "Social Conflict, Local Justice: Organizational Responses to the Astructural Bias." *Supplement to Interaction*, publication of the Network Interaction for Conflict Resolution, 4, no. 1 (Spring 1992): 1-4.

Moore, Christopher W. *The Mediation Process: Practical Strategies for Resolving Conflict*. San Francisco: Jossey-Bass Publishers, 1986.

Morrill, C. "The Private Ordering of Professional Relations." In *Hidden Conflict in Organizations: Uncovering Behind-the-Scenes Disputes*, 92-115. Ed. D. M. Kolb and J. M. Bartunek. Newbury Park, Calif.: Sage Publications, 1992.

Mulholland, Joan. *The Language of Negotiation: A Handbook of Practical Strategies for Improving Communication*. New York: Routledge, 1991.

Pike, Adele W. "Moral Outrage and Moral Discourse in Nurse–Physician Collaboration." *Journal of Professional Nursing* 7, no. 6 (November 1991): 351-363.

Pruitt, Dean G. *Negotiation Behavior*. New York: Academic Press, 1981.

Pruitt, Dean G., and Kenneth Kressel. "The Mediation of Social Conflict: An Introduction." *Journal of Social Issues* 41, no. 2 (1985): 1-10.

Raelin, J. A. *The Clash of Cultures: Managers and Professionals*. Harvard Business School Press: Boston, 1986.

Raiffa, Howard. *The Art and Science of Negotiation*. Cambridge: Harvard University Press, 1982.

Robbins, S. P. "'Conflict Management' and 'Conflict Resolution' Are Not Synonymous Terms." *California Management Review* 21, no. 2 (1978): 67-75.

Rogers, N. H., and C. A. McEwen. *Mediation: Law, Policy, Practice*. Rochester, N.Y.: The Lawyers Co-operative Publishing Co., 1989.

Schattschneider, H. J. "Power Relationships Between Physician and Nurse." *Humane Medicine* 6, no. 3 (1990): 197-201.

Schauer, F. "The Right to Die as a Case Study in Third-Order Decision Making." *The Journal of Medicine and Philosophy* 17 (1992): 573-587.

Sheppard, Blair H., Kathryn Blumenfeld-Jones and Jonelle Roth. "Informal Thirdpartyship: Studies of Everyday Conflict Intervention." In *Mediation Research: The Process and Effectiveness of Third-Party Intervention*, 166-189. Ed. Kenneth Kressel, Dean G. Pruitt and Associates. San Francisco: Jossey-Bass Publishers, 1989.

Sherif, M., et al. *Intergroup Conflict and Cooperation: The Robbers Cave Experiment*. Norman, Okla.: University of Oklahoma Book Exchange, 1961.

Shook, V., and N. Milner. "Thinking About Interdisciplinary Inquiry on Culture and Disputing." *Negotiation Journal* 5, no. 2 (1989): 134-147.

Slaikeu, Karl A. "Designing Dispute Resolution Systems in the Health Care Industry." *Negotiation Journal* 5, no. 4 (1989): 395-400.

Tjosvold, D. "Interdependence Approach to Conflict Management in Organizations." In *Managing Conflict: An Interdisciplinary Approach*, 41-50. Ed. M. A. Rahim. New York: Praeger, 1989.

—————. "The Goal Interdependence Approach to Communication in Conflict: An Organizational Study." In *Theory and Research in Conflict Management*, 15-27. Ed. M. A. Rahim. New York: Praeger, 1990.

Tranøy, K. E. "Biomedical Value Conflict." *Hastings Center Report* (August 1998): 8-10.

Ury, William L., Jeanne M. Brett and Stephen B. Goldberg. *Getting Disputes Resolved: Designing Systems to Cut the Costs of Conflict*. Jossey-Bass Publishers: San Francisco, 1988.

Victor, B., and J. B. Cullen. "The Organizational Bases of Ethical Work Climates." *Administrative Science Quarterly* 33, no. 1 (1988): 101-125.

Waldron, Edward E. "Ethics Committees, Decision-Making Quality Assurance, and Conflict Resolution." *The Journal of Clinical Ethics* 3, no. 4 (Winter 1992): 290-291.

Walker, R. M., S. H. Miles, C. B. Stocking and M. Siegler. "Physicians' and Nurses' Perceptions of Ethics Problems on General Medical Services." *Journal of General Intern Medicine* 6 (1991): 424-429.

West, Mary Beth. "Mediation and Communication Techniques in Ethics Consultation." *The Journal of Clinical Ethics* 3, no. 4 (Winter 1992): 291-292.

West, Mary Beth, and Joan McIver Gibson. "Facilitating Medical Ethics Case Review: What Ethics Committees Can Learn from Mediation and Facilitation Techniques." *Cambridge Quarterly on Healthcare Ethics* 1 (1992): 63-74.

Part 3

Chapter 9—Action Research on Ethical Deliberation

Billiet, J., et al. *Actes du colloque: Méthodologie et pratique de la recherche-action.* Brussels: Royaume de Belgique, Programme national de recherche en sciences sociales, 1980.

Colloque recherche action. Actes du Colloque recherche action, Université du Québec à Chicoutimi, 1981. Chicoutimi: Université du Québec à Chicoutimi, 1982.

Grand'Maison, Jacques, and Solange Lefebvre, eds. *Une génération bouc émissaires: Enquête sur les baby boomers,* 3ᵉ dossier de la recherche-action dans le diocèse Saint-Jérôme. Montreal: Fides, 1993.

————. eds. *La Part des aînées: Recherche-action.* 4ᵉ dossier. Montreal: Fides, 1994.

Holland, Joe, and Peter Henriot. *Social Analysis,* rev. ed. Maryknoll, N.Y.: Orbis/Center of Concern, 1984.

Nadeau, Jean-Guy, ed. "La Praxéologie pastorale: Orientations et parcours," vols. 1 and 2. *Cahiers d'études pastorales IV.* Montreal: Fides, 1987.

Walzer, Michael. *Spheres of Justice.* New York: Basic Books, 1983.

Winter, Gibson. *Elements for a Social Ethic.* New York: Macmillan, 1966.

————. *Liberating Creation.* New York: Crossroad, 1981.

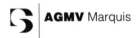

MEMBER OF THE SCABRINI GROUP

Quebec, Canada
2001